R. K. Weber, R. Keerl, S. D. Schaefer, R. C. Della Rocca (Eds.)

Atlas of Lacrimal Surgery

R.K. Weber R. Keerl S.D. Schaefer R.C. Della Rocca (Eds.)

Atlas of Lacrimal Surgery

With 232 Figures and 20 Tables

Springer

Rainer K. Weber, MD
Professor and Head
Division of Paranasal Sinus and Skull Base Surgery, Traumatology
Department of Otorhinolaryngology
Hospital Karlsruhe
Moltkestraße 90
D-76133 Karlsruhe, Germany
rainerweber@rainerweber.de

Rainer E. Keerl, MD
Assistant professor and Chief
Department of Otorhinolaryngology
St.-Elisabeth-Hospital
St.-Elisabeth-Straße 23
D-94315 Straubing, Germany
rainer.keerl@klinikum-straubing.de

Steven D. Schaefer, MD, FACS
Professor and Chair
Department of Otolaryngology
New York Eye and Ear Infirmary
New York Medical College
310 East 14th St.
New York, NY10003, USA
sschaefer@nyee.edu

Roberto C. Della Rocca, MD, FACS
Professor and Chief
Division of Oculoplastic and Orbital Surgery
New York Eye and Ear Infirmary
New York Medical College
Chairman
Department of Ophthalmology
St Luke's Roosevelt Hospital Center New York, NY
310 East 14th St.
New York, NY10003, USA
rdellaro@chpnet.org

Additional material to this book can be downloaded from http://extras.springer.com.

ISBN 978-3-662-50034-7 ISBN 978-3-540-68215-8 (eBook)
DOI 10.1007/978-3-540-68215-8

Springer is a part of Springer Science + Business Media
springer.com

Softcover reprint of the hardcover 1st edition 2007

Editor: Gabriele Schröder, Heidelberg, Germany
Desk Editor: Martina Himberger, Heidelberg, Germany
Cover design: Frido Steinen-Broo, eStudio Calamar, Spain
Reproduction and Typesetting: am-productions GmbH, Wiesloch, Germany
Production: LE-TEX Jelonek, Schmidt & Vöckler GbR, Leipzig, Germany

Printed on acid-free paper 27/3100 – YL – 5 4 3 2 1 0

Preface

To dry people's eyes – that's one of the great challenges in lacrimal surgery. Different localizations of the stenosis, lesions after tumor surgery or trauma, and epiphora in children or adults are different conditions that need various operative procedures to treat a patient individually and successfully.

The close relationship between the eyes and nose demands an interdisciplinary approach to lacrimal surgery. Therefore, ophthalmologists, otorhinolaryngologists as well as plastic surgeons are invited to contribute in solving a patient's problem.

This book is intended to serve as a practically oriented reference. In the first part, it contains chapters on pertinent surgical anatomy, physiology and pathophysiology as well as basic clinical and radiological evaluation. In the second part, well-known authorities from all over the world present their experience in all operative procedures currently available to dry patients' eyes. The accompanying DVD contains video clips of different operations highlighting key portions of these procedures.

I would like to express my gratitude to Springer, especially to Ms. Marion Philipp and Ms. Martina Himberger, and would also like to thank Alan Bellinger for reading and improving the manuscript. Additionally, I owe many thanks to my editorial colleagues, who did a great job working together on this book and to the authors who prepared excellent articles.

Finally, I wish all readers much pleasure while working through the chapters and hope that it helps them reach the goal of satisfied patients with dry eyes.

Rainer K. Weber

Contents

List of Contributors

S. Ahmad
Department of Ophthalmology
Oculoplastic and Orbital Surgery
New York Eye and Ear Infirmary/
St. Luke's – Roosevelt Hospital Center
New York, NY 10003, USA

I. Alobid
Department of ENT Hospital Clinic, Barcelona
University of Barcelona
08036 Barcelona, Spain
E-mail: 32874iao@comb.es

F. Ballesteros
Department of ENT Hospital Clinic, Barcelona
University of Barcelona
08036 Barcelona, Spain
E-mail: ferran.ballesteros@gmail.com

M. Bernal-Sprekelsen
Department of Otorhinolaryngology
Hospital Clinic, Barcelona
University of Barcelona
08036 Barcelona, Spain
E-mail: mbernal@clinic.ub.es

D. A. Della Rocca
Department of Ophthalmology
Oculoplastic and Orbital Surgery
New York Eye and Ear Infirmary/
St. Luke's – Roosevelt Hospital Center
New York, NY 10003, USA

R. C. Della Rocca
Department of Ophthalmology
Oculoplastic and Orbital Surgery
New York Eye and Ear Infirmary/
St. Luke's – Roosevelt Hospital Center
New York, NY 10003, USA
E-mail: rdellaro@chpnet.org

K.-H. Emmerich
Department of Ophthalmology
Hospital Darmstadt
Heidelberger Landstraße 379
64297 Darmstadt, Germany
E-mail: Augenklinik@Klinikum-Darmstadt.de

W. J. Heppt
Department of Otorhinolaryngology
Head and Neck Surgery
Hospital Karlsruhe
Moltkestraße 90
76133 Karlsruhe, Germany
E-mail: HNOKlinik@klinikum-karlsruhe.com

N. Jones
Department of Otorhinolaryngology
Head and Neck Surgery
Queen's Medical Centre
University Hospital
Nottingham NG7 2UH, UK
E-mail: Nick.Jones@nottingham.ac.uk

R. Keerl
Department of Otorhinolaryngology
St. Elisabeth Hospital Straubing
St.-Elisabeth-Straße 23
94315 Straubing, Germany
E-mail: keerlr@klinikum-straubing.de

P. Komínek
Clinic of Otorhinolaryngology
Faculty Hospital
Tr.17. Iistopadu Str. 1790
70852 Ostrava-Poruba, Czech Republic
E-mail: kominek@nemfm.cz

H.-W. Meyer-Rüsenberg
Department of Ophthalmology
St.-Josefs-Hospital Hagen
University of Hagen
Dreieckstraße 17
58097 Hagen, Germany
E-mail: info@kkh-hagen.de

S. Mirza
Department of Otorhinolaryngology
Head and Neck Surgery
Queen's Medical Centre
University Hospital
Nottingham NG7 2UH, UK

J. Mullol Miret
Department of ENT Hospital Clinic, Barcelona
University of Barcelona
08036 Barcelona, Spain

F. Paulsen
Department of Anatomy and Cell Biology
Martin Luther University of Halle-Wittenberg
Große Steinstraße 52
06097 Halle (Saale), Germany
E-mail: friedrich.paulsen@medizin.uni-halle.de

L. Pierroth
Oculoplastic and Orbital Surgery
Ophthalmic Hospital Dardenne
Bonn, Germany

P. Preechawi
Department of Ophthalmology
Oculoplastic and Orbital Surgery
New York Eye and Ear Infirmary/
St. Luke's – Roosevelt Hospital Center
New York, NY 10003, USA

S. Rosenbaum
Department of Ophthalmology
New York Eye and Ear Infirmary/
St. Luke's – Roosevelt Hospital Center
New York, NY 10003, USA

S. D. Schaefer
Department of Otolaryngology
and Communicative Sciences
New York Eye and Ear Infirmary/
New York Medical College
310 East 14th Street
New York, NY 10003, USA
E-mail: sschaefer@nyee.edu

M. Tomás-Barberán
University Hospital Son Dureta
07014 Palma de Mallorca, Spain
E-mail: mtomas@hsd.es

R. Ungerechts
Department of Ophthalmology
Hospital Darmstadt
Heidelberger Landstraße 379
64297 Darmstadt, Germany

R. K. Weber
Division of Paranasal Sinus
and Skull Base Surgery, Traumatology
Department of Otorhinolaryngology
Hospital Karlsruhe
Moltkestraße 90
76133 Karlsruhe, Germany
rainerweber@rainerweber.de

K. Wilhelm
Department of Radiology
University Hospital Bonn
Sigmund-Freud-Straße 25
53127 Bonn, Germany
E-mail: wilhelm@uni-bonn.de

Chapter 1

Anatomy and Physiology of the Nasolacrimal Ducts

1

Friedrich Paulsen

Core Messages

- The tear film is produced by the lacrimal gland and the different structures of the eye lid. Its composition is controlled by the lacrimal functional unit.
- The ocular surface epithelia together with the lacrimal gland produce a unique subset of membrane bound and secretory mucins that stabilize the tear film, fix it to the epithelia, support binding of bacteria, and are of great importance to tear physiology.
- TFF peptides TFF1 and TFF3 of conjunctival origin influence the rheological properties of the tear film.
- Drainage of tears involves a number of different mechanisms; of these the action of the lacrimal part of the orbicularis oculi muscle is most important to bring tear fluid into the lacrimal sac. Epithelial secretion products, the surrounding cavernous body, and the arrangement of connective tissue fibers are most important to drain lacrimal fluid from the lacrimal sac into the inferior meatus of the nose.
- The epithelium of the nasolacrimal ducts eases tear flow by the production of mucins and TFF peptides. Moreover, it contributes to antimicrobial defense and is able to absorb tear fluid components.
- The lacrimal sac and nasolacrimal duct are surrounded by a cavernous body. While regulating the blood flow, the specialized blood vessels permit opening and closing of the lumen of the lacrimal passage affected by the bulging and subsiding of the cavernous body, while at the same time regulating tear outflow. The blood vessels are connected to the vessels of the outer eye and could act as a feedback signal for tear-fluid production.

Contents

1.1 Introduction

Study of the nasolacrimal ducts is a synthesis of two disciplines, ophthalmology and otorhinolaryngology, which work closely together in the treatment of naso-lacrimal disorders. During recent years a bulk of new diagnostic and therapeutic methods, such as nasolacrimal endoscopy, laser-assisted dacryocystorhinostomy, transcanalicular surgery, and interventional radiological therapies, have been applied to the nasolacrimal system; however, common knowledge about anatomy and physiology of the nasolacrimal ducts, and of tear flow through the nasolacrimal passage, is not well developed.

This chapter summarizes recent advances in knowledge of the nasolacrimal ducts and discusses them in conjunction with nasolacrimal duct physiology.

1.2 Anatomy and Physiology of the Ocular Surface and Adnexa

To understand the physiology of tear flow through the nasolacrimal passage, and also its pathophysiology (Chap. 2), basic knowledge of the whole lacrimal system is necessary. The ocular surface and its adnexa comprise the cornea, the conjunctiva with bulbar, fornical and palpebral parts, the main lacrimal gland, and the glands of the eye lids, i.e., Meibomian, Moll, Zeis, and accessory lacrimal glands as well as the nasolacrimal system; the latter consists of the upper and lower puncta, the paired lacrimal canaliculi, the lacrimal sac, and the nasolacrimal duct (Fig. 1.1). The nasolacrimal ducts collect the tear fluid from the ocular surface and convey it into the nasal cavity, whereas all other structures contribute to formation of the preocular and cornea tear film. The tear film serves to protect and lubricate the ocular surface, allowing for protection of the cornea and consistent clarity of vision.

The preocular tear film contains water, protective antimicrobials, cytokines, lipids, and mucins, and is divided into three components: a lipid, an aqueous, and a mucus component. The lipid component is secreted by the Meibomian glands in the eyelid and forms the superficial layer of the tear film (Fig. 1.2). The aqueous component contains electrolytes, water, and a large variety of proteins, peptides, and glycopeptides, and is secreted primarily by the lacrimal gland as well as the accessory lacrimal glands (glands of Krause, glands of Wolfring) of the lids (Fig. 1.2). The mucus component is the product of conjunctival goblet and epithelial cells, corneal epithelial cells [4], and acinar as well as excretory duct cells of the lacri-

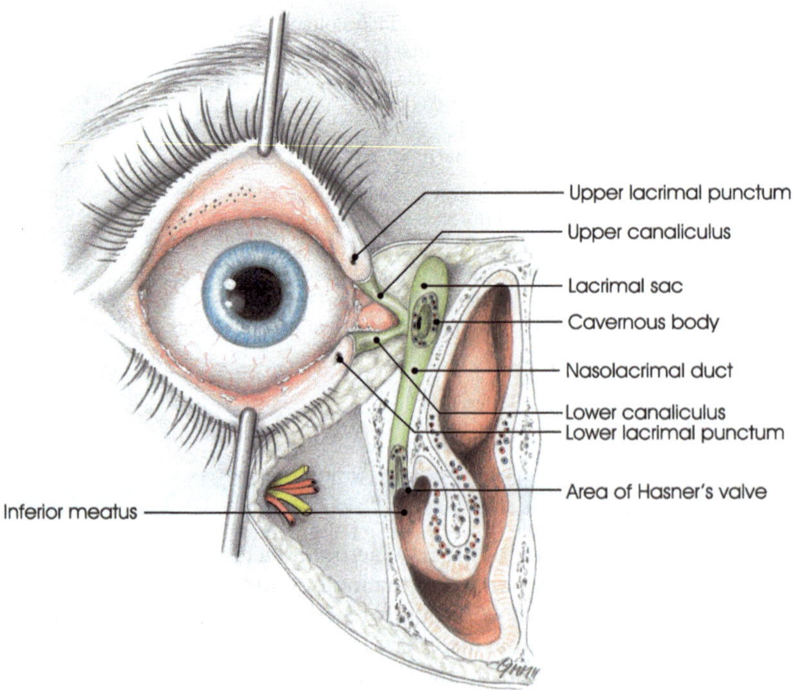

Fig. 1.1. Ocular surface and nasolacrimal ducts. The ocular bulbus with cornea and bulbar conjunctiva, as well as tarsal conjunctiva, are visible. At the medial rim of the upper and lower lid open the lacrimal puncta leading into the lacrimal sac via the upper and lower canaliculi. The lacrimal sac is situated in the orbital lacrimal fossa and proceeds into the nasolacrimal duct. The nasolacrimal duct is surrounded by a bony canal created by the maxillary and lacrimal bones and opens into the inferior meatus of the nose. Both lacrimal sac and nasolacrimal duct are surrounded by a vascular plexus comparable to a cavernous body that is connected to the cavernous system of the nose. (From [26])

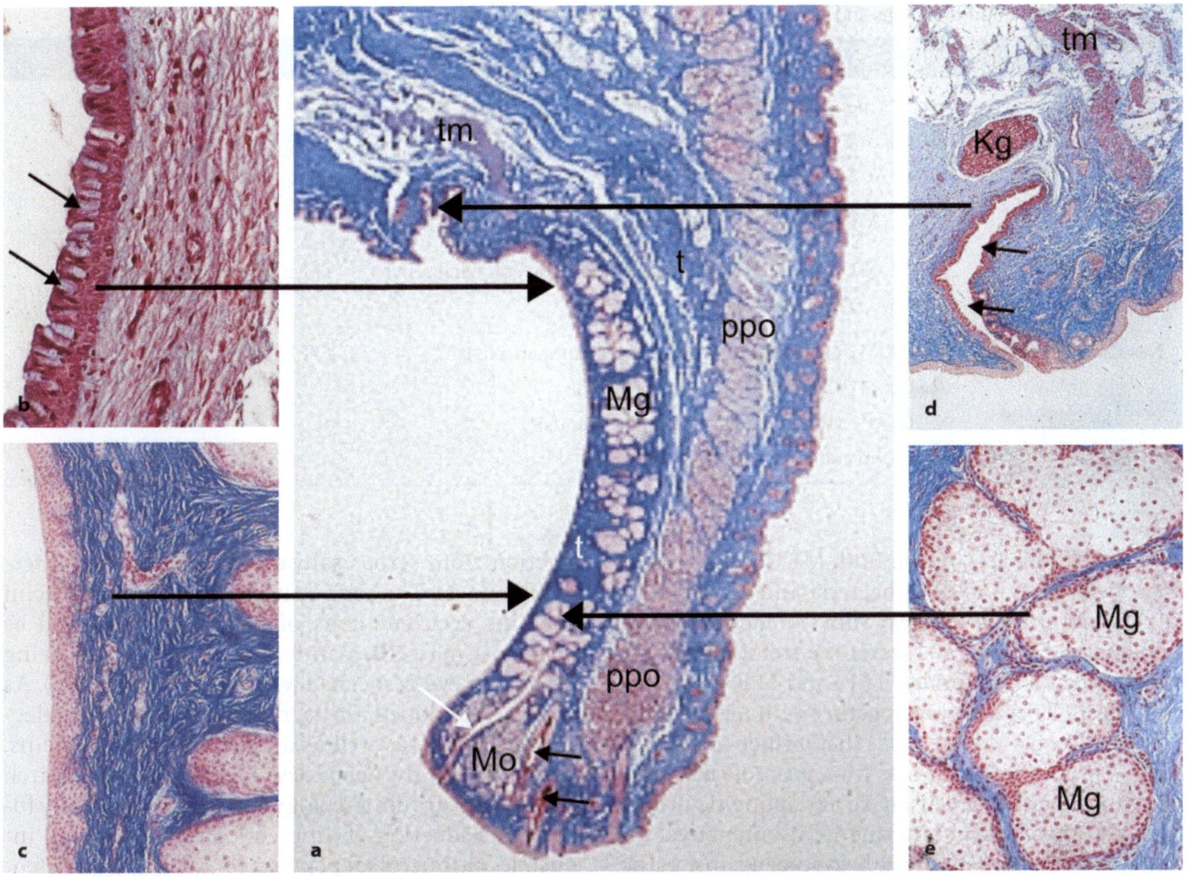

Fig. 1.2. Structures of the eyelid. **a** Overview. Sagittal section through an eye lid. *tm* tarsalis muscle, *t* tarsus, *ppo* palpebral part of orbicularis muscle, *Mg* Meibomian gland. *White arrow:* excretory duct of Meibomian gland; *Mo* Moll's gland. *Black arrows:* sections through eyelashes. **b–e** Representative magnifications of the areas marked by a *large black arrow* in **a**. **b** Conjunctival epithelium in the area of the tarsal plate near the fornix. The epithelium consists of columnar epithelial cells with integrated goblet cells (*arrows*). Tight connective tissue of the tarsus underlies the epithelium. **c** Conjunctival epithelium in the area of the tasal plate near the rim of the eye lid. A non-cornified squamous epithelium covers the underlying tarsal plate. Parts of the Meibomian gland are visible. **d** The magnification shows an accessory lacrimal gland (Krause's gland; *Kg*). A small excretory duct opens into an infolding of the fornical conjunctiva (*arrows*). Above the gland parts of the tarsalis muscle (*tm*) are visible. **e** Magnification of a part of a Meibomian gland (*Mg*) reveals its sebaceous character. The gland is embedded in the tarsal plate. (Figure 2 a is from [27], Figures 2 b–e are from [6])

mal gland, which have recently been shown to produce mucins (Fig. 1.2) [10, 16]. The mucinous layer helps to spread the lipid and aqueous layer across the cornea.

1.2.1 Ocular Surface

The surfaces of the ocular epithelia, both corneal and conjunctival, provide a specialized and important interface between the tear fluid and the epithelium that stabilizes the fluid layer. That interface includes the undulating membrane ridges on the apical cell's apical membrane, termed microplicae, and emanating from their apices, a layer termed the glycocalyx. Membrane bound mucins (MUCs 1, 4, and 16) of corneal and conjunctival epithelial cells are present in the glycocalyx layer. Soluble mucins (MUC5AC) from conjunctival goblet cells, as well as MUC5B and MUC7 from lacrimal glands, are in solution in the

Table 1.1. Distribution of mucins and TFF peptides in the healthy lacrimal system

Localization	Mucins	TFF peptides
Lacrimal gland	MUC1 (membrane bound on acinar cells) MUC4, MUC5B, MUC7 (in acinar cells) MUC5AC (in excretory duct cells)	
Cornea	MUC1, MUC4, MUC16 (membrane bound on epithelial cells)	
Conjunctiva	MUC1, MUC4, MUC16 (membrane bound on epithelial cells) MUC5AC (in goblet cells)	TFF1, TFF3 (in goblet cells)
Nasolacrimal ducts	MUC1, MUC4 (membrane bound on columnar cells) MUC2, MUC5AC, MUC5B (in goblet cells) MUC5AC, MUC5B (in intraepithelial glands) MUC7 (in columnar cells)	TFF1 (goblet cell associated); TFF3 (in columnar cells)

tear film (Table 1.1) [4, 10]. Both MUC5B and MUC7 have been shown to bind bacteria and contribute to innate immunity of the tear film. Besides MUC5AC, conjunctival goblet cells secret the trefoil family factor peptides (TFF peptides) TFF1 and TFF3 (Table 1.1) [6]. The TFF peptides are, together with mucins, typical constituents of mucus gels that influence the rheological properties of the tear film, promote migration of corneal epithelial cells, have antiapoptotic properties, and induce cell scattering [5]. Conjunctival and corneal epithelial cells are able to react against pathogens by the production of inducible antimicrobial peptides (a kind of body-own antibiotics). In addition, in certain disease states the corneal cells are able to produce TFF3.

1.2.2 Lacrimal Gland

The lacrimal gland is anterior in the superolateral region of the orbit, and is divided into two parts by the levator palpebrae superioris muscle, the anterior palpebral segment, and orbital portion of the gland. The lacrimal gland consists of acini that consist of a luminar lining of columnar epithelial cells that are surrounded by a basal layer of myoepithelial cells and an enclosing basement membrane. The human lacrimal gland is a tubulo-alveolar gland of serous type. Intercalated and 6–12 interlobular ducts drain the secretions into the conjunctival fornix beneath the temporal bone. The tubules discharge without any characteristic excretory duct system (histological distinction from serous salivary glands) into the interlobular ducts. The connective tissue between the acini contains accumulations of lymphocytes as well as many plasma cells mainly secreting IgA and being part of the eye-associated lymphoid tissue (EALT). As already mentioned, the lacrimal gland produces electrolytes, water, as well as a large variety of proteins, peptides, and glycopeptides; of these, recent research regarding tear film rheology and innate immunity focus on production of different constitutively and inducible antimicrobial peptides [8], such as beta defensins, surfactant proteins A and D [1], as well as mucins MUC4, MUC5AC, MUC5B, and MUC7 which are secreted by the lacrimal gland into the tear film (Table 1.1) [10, 16].

1.2.3 Eyelid

The "skeleton" of the eyelid is a collagen plate called the tarsus (Fig. 1.2). It contains a row of branched alveolar sebaceous glands, unrelated to the eyelashes. These tarsal or Meibomian glands have punctated openings along the free edge of the eyelid close to its posteroir margin. They produce a lipid material whose synthesis is dependent on neuronal, hormonal, and vascular factors [7]. This lipid material is fluid, spreads easily, is a surfactant as well as an aqueous barrier, and must remain functional after a blink. To satisfy these requirements, the Meibomian lipids have a specific composition. Even after delivery, it may be modified by lipases produced by ocular bacteria, and

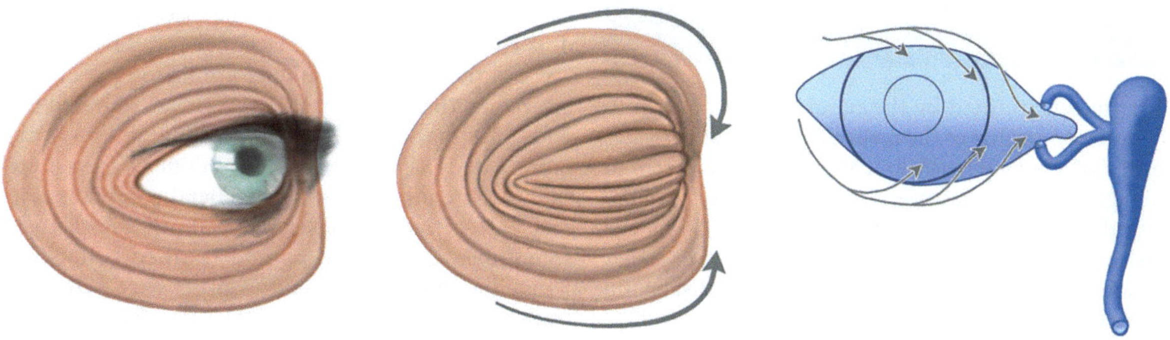

Fig. 1.3. The action of the palpebral part of the orbicularis eye muscle and resulting tear-film dynamics. Lid closure leads to a time shifted contraction of the orbicularis eye muscle from temporally to nasally at the same time moving the tear film to the medial cantal region

modifications in the lipid components can lead to unique disease states. Sexual hormones, especially androgens, seem to play a decisive role in Meibomian physiology [24].

Near the anterior margin of the eye lids there are two or three rows of cilia – the eyelashes (Fig. 1.2). In the middle of the lid is the cross-striated orbicularis oculi muscle. The fiber bundles of its palpebral part overlap one another like tiles on a roof. Orbicularis action is triggered by the facial nerve leading to time-shifted lid closure from temporally to nasally and at the same time moving the tears to the medial cantal region and "lacrimal lake" (Fig. 1.3). The tendon of the cross-striated levator palpebral muscle is inserted into anterior one-third of the tarsus with extension to the skin layer to help define the eyelid crease. The smooth tarsalis muscle originates and lies on the posterior surface of the levator muscle and inserts into the superior tarsal margin. The tone of the latter muscle is determined by autonomic nervous supply, and responds to neosynephrine stimulation. This contributes to the elevation of the upper eyelid. Its action is specifically demonstrated with retraction of the upper eyelid associated with thyroid eye disease. The apocrine ciliary glands (Moll's glands) open close to the eyelashes. These apocrine glands are active from birth, in producing agents against pathogenic microorganisms in the eyelid shaft and on the ocular surface, i.e., lysozyme, beta-defensin-2, adrenomedullin, lactoferrin, and IgA [23]. In the conjunctival fornix the eyelid also contains small accessory lacrimal glands (Krause's glands, Wolfring's glands; Fig. 1.2). Although much smaller, these glands are histologically comparable to the main lacrimal gland. They contribute to the tear film as basal aqueous secretors.

1.2.4 The Lacrimal Functional Unit

The cornea possesses the richest sensory innervation of the body to detect noxious stimuli. The trigeminal sensory neurons (CN V) that innervate the eye vary in their chemical composition and electrophysiological properties, and can be classified according to the stimuli that activate them preferentially: mechanical forces; temperature; or irritant chemicals. Different classes of noxious stimuli (mechanical injuries, heat, extreme cold) activate the population of sensory fibers of the ocular surface to a different degree and evoke unpleasant sensations of distinct quality [3].

It is recognized that the tear film is secreted reflexively by the "lacrimal functional unit" which is composed of the ocular surface tissues (cornea and conjunctiva, including goblet cells and Meibomian glands), the lacrimal glands (main and accessory), and their interconnecting sensory (CN V) and autonomic (CN VII) innervation. This reflex secretion is initiated by subconscious stimulation of the highly innervated ocular surface epithelia [22]. The human nasolacrimal ducts are integrated in this reflex arc, as shown below.

1.3 Anatomy and Physiology of the Nasolacrimal Ducts

Tear fluid is drained by the nasolacrimal ducts into the inferior meatus of the nose. The lacrimal passages consist of a bony passage and a membranous lacrimal passage. The bony passage is formed anteriorly by the frontal process of the maxilla and posteriorly by the lacrimal bone. The membranous lacrimal passages include the lacrimal canaliculi, the lacrimal sac, and the nasolacrimal duct (Figs. 1.1, 1.4).

The upper and lower canaliculi are lined by pseudostratified and stratified columnar epithelium and are surrounded by a dense ring of connective tissue, as well as by muscle fibers of the lacrimal portion of the orbicularis oculi muscle (Horner's muscle), which surrounds the deep portion of the medial canthal tendon and the dome of the lacrimal sac. The lacrimal sac and the nasolacrimal duct are lined by a double-layered epithelium (Fig. 1.5) and are surrounded by a wide ranging vascular system comparable to a cavernous body (Figs. 1.1, 1.6). The double-layered epithelium is composed of a superficial columnar layer and a deep flattened layer of basal cells. Both layers sometimes appear as a pseudostratified epithelium. Kinociliae-lining single epithelial cells are a common finding in the lower part of the nasolacrimal duct (Fig. 2.1); however, most epithelial cells are lined by microvilli (Fig. 1.5). In addition to the epithelial cells, goblet cells are integrated in the epithelium as single cells or form characteristic intraepithelial mucous glands (Fig. 1.5) [9].

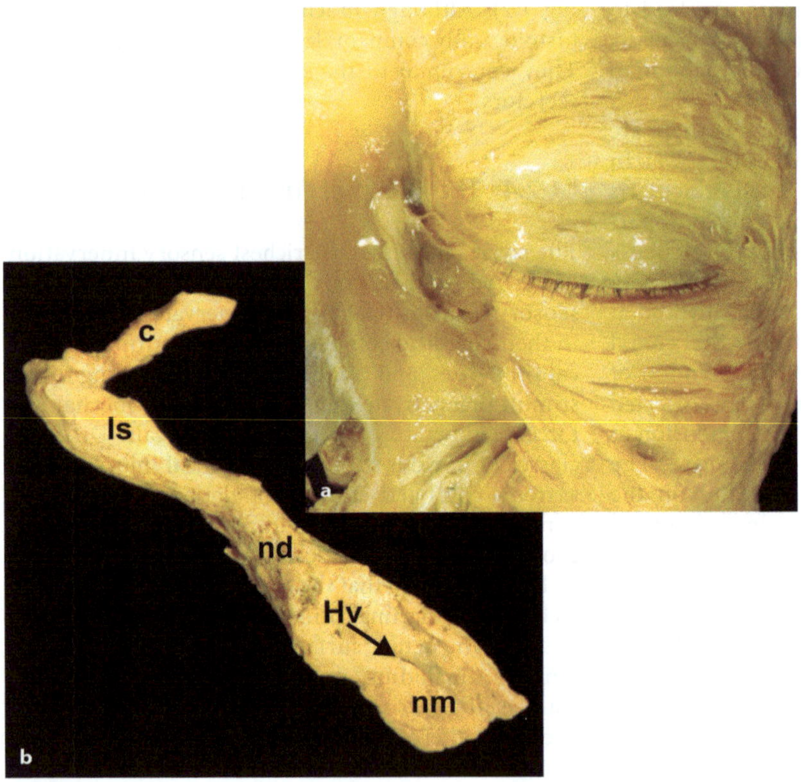

Fig. 1.4. Macroscopy of the nasolacrimal ducts. **a** View of a prepared lacrimal system in situ (Anatomical collection of the Christian Albrecht University of Kiel, Germany). **b** Macroscopic view of a prepared nasolacrimal system removed from its bony canal. *c* Lacrimal canaliculi (individual canaliculi not distinguishable), *ls* lacrimal sac, *nd* nasolacrimal duct, *nm* mucous membrane of the nose, *hv* area of Hasner's valve opening of the nasolacrimal duct into inferior meatus of the nose. (From [10])

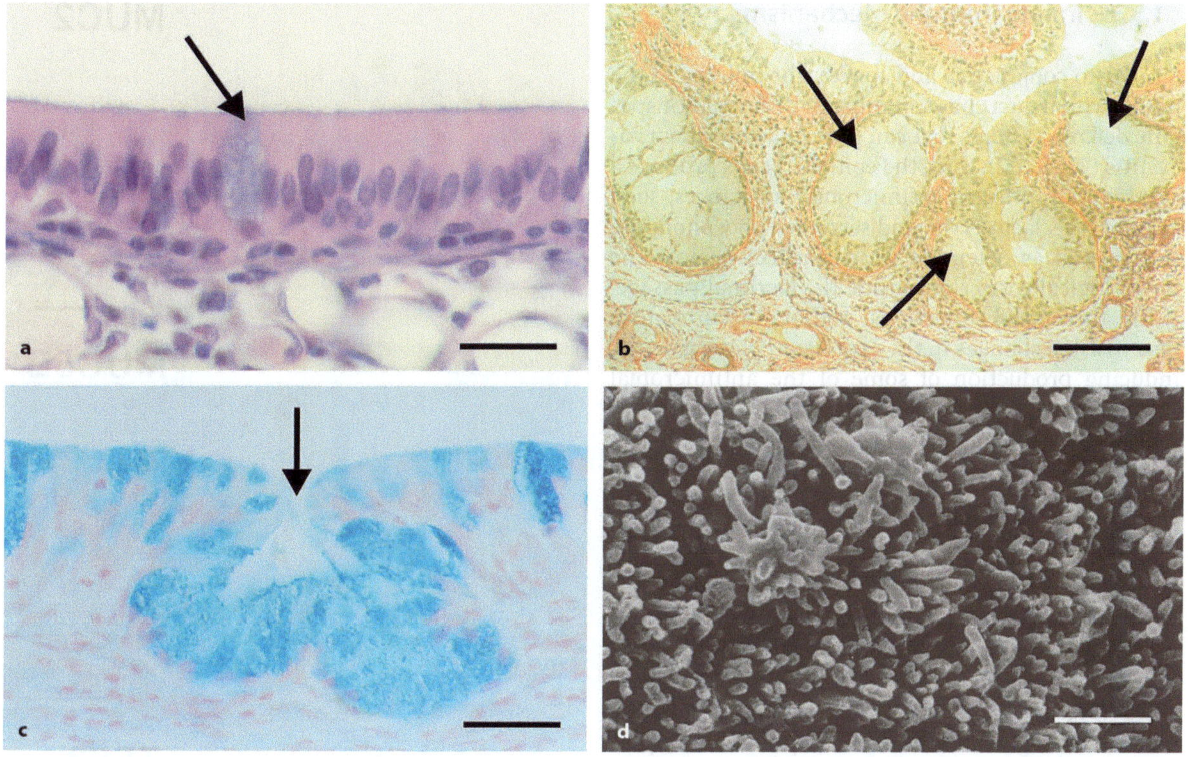

Fig. 1.5. Light microscopy and scanning electron microscopy (SEM) of the lining epithelium of the nasolacrimal ducts. **a** Epithelium of the nasolacrimal duct consisting of a basal cell layer and a superficial columnar layer. A single goblet cell is integrated in the epithelium (*arrow*). Bar=42 µm. **b** Goblet cells show a characteristic arrangement of several cell groups in the upper part of the lacrimal sac forming mucous glands (*arrows*). Resorcin–fuchsine–thiazine picric-acid staining, bar=84 µm **c** Goblet cells form a mucous gland that lies in the lamina propria and has its own secretory duct (*arrow*). Alcian blue staining (pH 1); bar=27 µm **d** An SEM micrograph of the surface of epithelial cells in the lacrimal sac. The SEM reveals a surface covering of epithelial cells by a trimming with microvilli. (From [10])

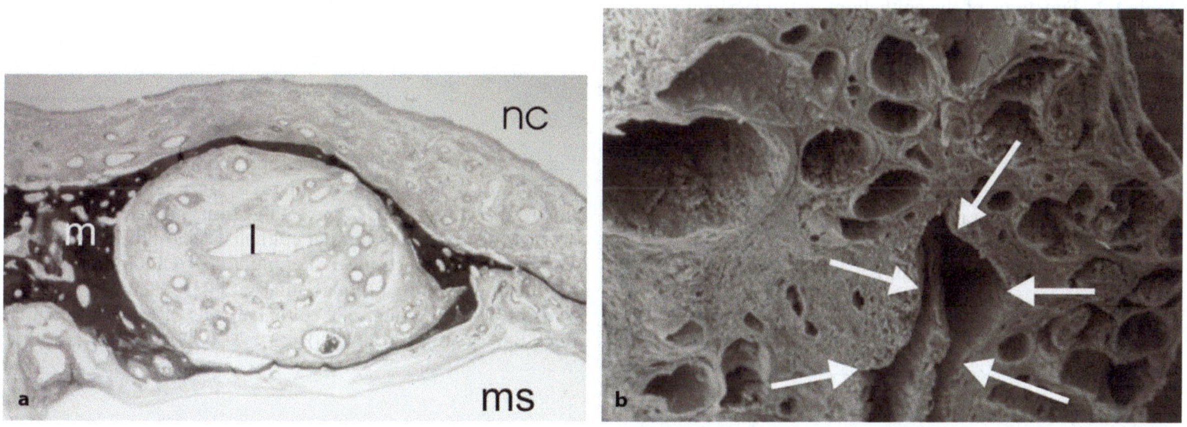

Fig. 1.6. The vascular system of the nasolacrimal ducts. **a** Cross-section through the nasolacrimal duct with azan staining. More than two-thirds of the surrounding bony canal is filled by vascular plexus. *m* maxillary bone, *l* lumen of the nasolacrimal duct, *nc* nasal cavity, *ms* maxillary sinus. **b** Scanning electron microscopic photograph of a horizontally sectioned lacrimal system. Wide-luminated blood vessels surround the lumen (*arrows*) of the nasolacrimal passage. (From [10])

1.3.1 Innate Immune Mechanisms

Similar to conjunctiva and cornea, the mucosa of the nasolacrimal ducts has a number of different nonspecific defense systems that can protect against dacryocystitis (Table 1.2); thus, the epithelial cells produce a spectrum of different antimicrobial substances, such as lysozyme, lactoferrin, and secretory phospholipase A2, as well as defensins which protect against the physiological germ flora inside the lacrimal passage. With threatened infectious and/or inflammatory dacryosistis, changes in the expression pattern occur, inducing production of some of the antimicrobial substances, e.g., antimicrobial peptides, such as human inducible beta defensins 2 and 3, which are not produced under healthy conditions [18].

The secretory product of the mucus component formed by goblet cells and epithelial cells has been attributed largely to immunological response. It contains mucins MUC1, MUC2, MUC4, MUC5AC, MUC5B, and MUC7 (Fig. 1.7; Table 1.2) [11]. Furthermore, the epithelium of the nasolacrimal ducts expresses and produces the TFF peptides TFF1 and TFF3 (Fig. 1.7; Table 1.2) [15]. Disturbances in the balance of single mucins or TFF-peptides are important in the development of dacryostenosis, dacryolithiasis, and dacryocystitis (see Chap. 2). Mucins have several functions. In addition to lubricating the mucosa and "water-proofing" to regulate epithelial cell hydration, mucins protect mucosal surfaces against potentially harmful substances; however, a variety of

Table 1.2. Functions of the epithelium of the lacrimal sac and nasolacrimal duct

Secretion of antimicrobial substances (lysozyme, lactoferrin, secretory phospholipase A_2, bactericidal-permeability-increasing protein, heparin-binding protein, human β-defensins, surfactant proteins)
Secretion of mucins (MUC2, MUC5AC, MUC5B, MUC7), production of membrane-bound mucins (MUC1, MUC4, MUC16)
Secretion of TFF peptides (TFF1, TFF3)
Production of lipids
Absorption of tear-fluid components

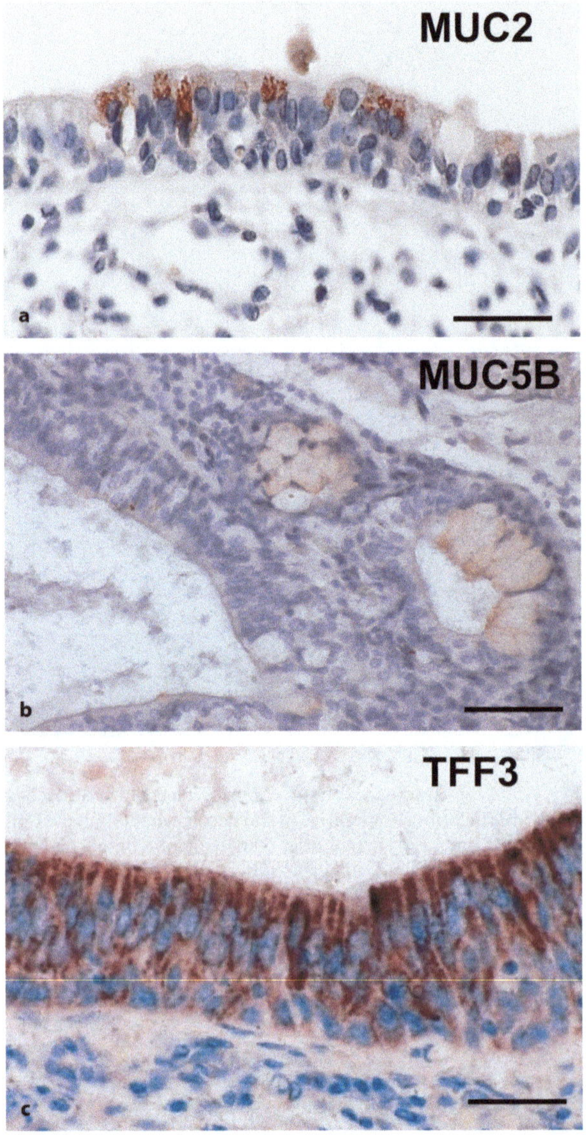

Fig. 1.7. Distribution of mucins and trefoil factor family (TFF) peptides in the epithelium of the nasolacrimal ducts. **a** Detection (*red*) of mucin MUC2 revealing strong supranuclear granular staining in single columnar epithelial cells of the lacrimal sac. Bar=56 μm. **b** Detection (*red*) of mucin MUC5B in intraepithelial mucous glands of the lacrimal sac. Bar=38 μm **c** Detection (*red*) of TFF3 in columnar epithelial cells of the nasolacrimal duct. Bar=56 μm. (From [11])

oral and intestinal bacteria have been shown to produce sialidase, an enzyme that can degrade mucins by removing sialic acid. Additionally, oral and intestinal bacteria synthesize an array of other glycosidases which can attack the oligosaccharide residues of mucins [21]. Early results of current investigations reveal that such glycosidases are also present at the ocular surface.

Finally, secretory IgA (sIgA) is incorporated into the mucus layer of mucosal surfaces, supplementing the protective activity. It can interact with functionally diverse cells, including epithelial cells, B- and T-lymphocytes, NK cells, cells of the monocyte/macrophage lineage, and neutrophils [21]. All of these latter cell types, as well as sIgA, are present on, and in, the nasolacrimal ducts and belong to the lacrimal mucosal immune system (see below).

1.3.2 Adaptive Immune Mechanisms

Subepithelially, lymphocytes and other defense cells are amply present inside the efferent tear ducts, sometimes aggregated into follicles (Fig. 1.8). Aggregated follicles are present in nearly a third of nasolacrimal ducts from unselected cadavers with no known history of disease involving the eye, efferent tear ducts, or the nose. These aggregations and the surrounding tissue fulfill the criteria for designation as mucosa-associated lymphoid tissue (MALT). They consist of organized mucosal lymphoid tissue characterized by the presence of reactive germinal centers and mantle zones. Around the mantle zone there is an additional zone of somewhat larger cells corresponding to marginal zone cells. These larger cells extend into the overlying epithelium, forming a lymphoepithelium.

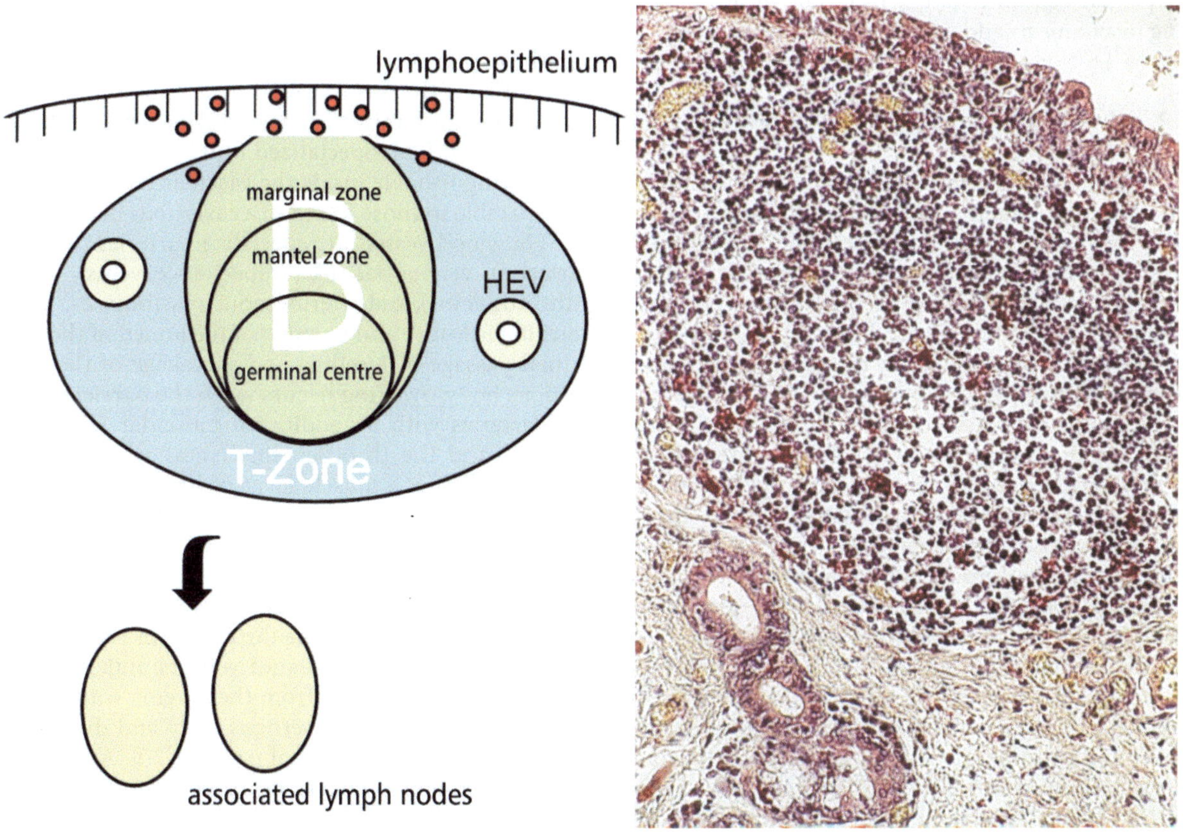

Fig. 1.8. Immunohistochemistry (*right*) and schematic drawing (*left*) of tear duct-associated lymphoid tissue (TALT). The TALT reveals a well-developed germinal center, a surrounding mantle zone, a marginal zone, and an overlying lymphoepithelium. The follicle is surrounded by a T-cell zone with high endothelial venules (HEV) for the entrance of immune cells. Moreover, per definition mucosa-associated lymphoid tissue (MALT) comprises also an associated lymph node region. (From [10])

1

In accordance with the terminology of MALT in other body regions, MALT of the human nasolacrimal ducts was termed TALT (Fig. 1.8) [17].

Specific secretory immunity depends on a sophisticated cooperation between the mucosal B-cell system and an epithelial glycoprotein called the *secretory component*. Initial stimulation of Ig-producing B-cells is believed to occur mainly in organized MALT. It has become evident that considerable regionalization or compartmentalization exists in MALT, perhaps being determined by different cellular expression profiles of adhesion molecules and/or the local antigenic repertoire. Antigenic stimulation of B cells results in the generation of predominantly IgA-synthesizing blasts that leave the mucosae via efferent lymphatics, pass through the associated lymph nodes into the thoracic duct, and enter the circulation. The cells then return selectively to the lamina propria (nasolacrimal ducts) as plasma cells or memory B cells by means of homing mechanisms and contribute to mucosal sIgA.

1.3.3 Mechanisms of Tear Drainage

Drainage of tears involves a number of different mechanisms (Table 1.3). Physical factors, such as gravity, respiration, and evaporation, have been suggested. A decisive role is played by capillary attraction, aided by contraction of the lacrimal portion of the orbicularis muscle with blinking, as well as distension of the lacrimal sac by the action of the orbicularis muscle [19].

The mucin diversity of the epithelium of the nasolacrimal ducts together with TFF peptides that are able to influence the rheological properties of tear fluid have already been mentioned. Besides antimicrobial defense, these components are necessary epithelial secretion products to enhance tear transport [12]. Disorders in the balance of single mucins and TFF peptides are described in Chap. 2.

The lamina propria of the lacrimal sac and nasolacrimal duct consist of two strata: underneath the epithelium, loose connective tissue containing a thin layer of elastic fibers and many lymphatic cells, sometimes arranged in follicles, as well as a rich venous plexus situated under the loose connective tissue that is connected caudally with the cavernous body of the nasal inferior turbinate. Collagen bundles and elastic and reticular fibers between the blood vessels of the rich venous plexus are arranged in a helical pattern

Table 1.3. Mechanisms of tear drainage

Active lacrimal pump mechanism aided by contraction of the lacrimal portion of the orbicularis muscle
Distension of the lacrimal sac by the action of the lacrimal portion of the orbicularis muscle
Epithelial secretion products (mucins and TFF peptides) of the epithelium of the lacrimal sac and nasolacrimal duct
"Wringing-out" mechanism governed by a system of helically arranged fibrillar structures
Opening and closing of the lumen of the lacrimal passage effected by the bulging and subsiding of the cavernous body
Capillarity
Respiration
Evaporation
Absorption of tear fluid through the lining epithelium of the lacrimal sac and nasolacrimal duct

and run spirally from the fornix of the lacrimal sac to the outlet of the nasolacrimal duct, where they contribute biomechanically to tear outflow during blinking (Fig. 1.9) [25]. Specialized types of blood vessels are distinguishable inside the vascular tissue and are comparable to those found in a cavernous body [20].

The blood vessels are specialized arteries (barrier arteries), venous lacunae (capacitance veins), veins (throttle veins), and arteriovenous anastomoses. They facilitate closure and opening of the lumen of the lacrimal passage by swelling and shrinkage of the cavernous body. Swelling occurs when the barrier arteries (arteries with an additional muscular layer) are opened and the throttle veins (veins whose tunica media contains a muscle layer of helically arranged smooth muscle cells) are closed. Filling of the capacitance veins (widely convoluted venous lacunae) occurs at the same time as closure of the lumen of the lacrimal passage. In contrast, closure of the barrier arteries and opening of the throttle veins reduces the blood flow to the capacitance veins, simultaneously allowing blood outflow from these veins with resultant shrinkage of the cavernous body and dilatation of the lumen of the lacrimal passage [20]. Arteriovenous anastomoses enable for direct blood flow between arteries and venous lacunae; thus, the subepithelially located capillary network can be avoided, and rapid filling of capacitance veins is possible when the shunts of the arteriovenous anastomoses are open. While regulating the blood flow, the specialized blood

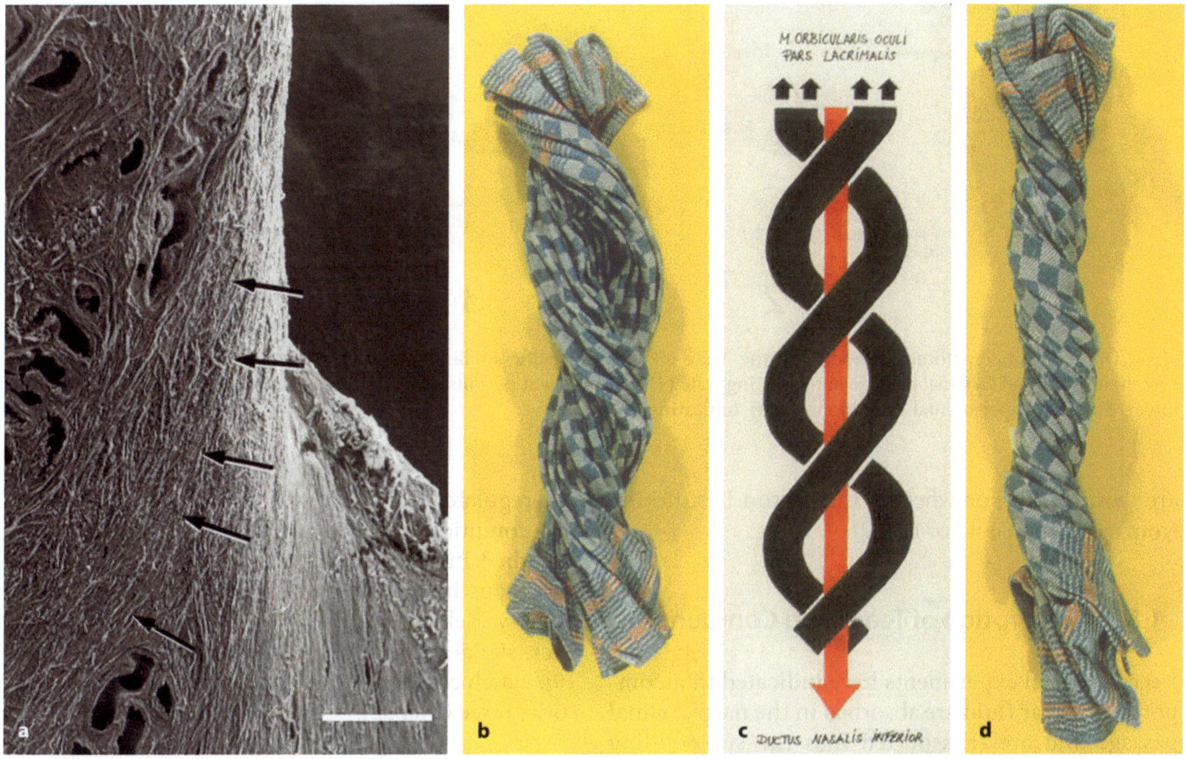

Fig. 1.9. Fibrillar structures of the nasolacrimal ducts. **a** Scanning electron microscopic photograph of the outer surface of a nasolacrimal duct revealing the helical arrangement of collagen fibrils (*arrows*). Bar=550 μm. **b–d** The arrangement of collagen and elastic fibers in a schematic view. If the nasolacrimal duct distends while blinking, it will be "wrung out" due to the screw-shaped arrangement of the collagen bundles. (From [10])

vessels permit opening and closing of the lumen of the lacrimal passage, effected by the bulging and subsiding of the cavernous body, and, at the same time, regulate tear outflow [20].

The presence of the cavernous body is lacking in nearly all textbooks of anatomy (Fig. 1.1) and is therefore unknown to most nasolacrimal surgeons as well as radiologists; however, it is densely innervated [14]. Epiphora related to emotions such as sorrow or happiness occur not only by increased tear secretion from the lacrimal gland and accessory lacrimal glands, but also by closure of the lacrimal passage. This mechanism acts, for example, to provide protection against foreign bodies that have entered the conjunctival sac: Not only is tear fluid production increased, but tear outflow is also interrupted by the swelling of the cavernous body to flush out the foreign body and protect the efferent tear ducts themselves [2, 14, 20]. Moreover, it can be assumed that the valves in the lacrimal sac and nasolacrimal duct described in the past by Rosenmüller, Hanske, Aubaret, Béraud, Krause, and Taillefer could be caused by different swelling states of the cavernous body and must therefore be considered as speculation [20].

The cavernous body of the efferent tear ducts actually plays an important role in the physiology of tear outflow regulation and can be influenced pharmacologically (Fig. 1.10) [2]. Interestingly, administration of a decongestant drug or insertion of a foreign body at the ocular surface both prolong the tear transit time significantly, but by different mechanisms. Application of a decongestant drug simultaneously with insertion of a foreign body shortens the tear transit time significantly compared to the effect of the decongestant drug alone, but there is no significant difference compared with application of a foreign body alone. The tear transit time is independent of the side (right or left) and gender, and whether the eyeglasses

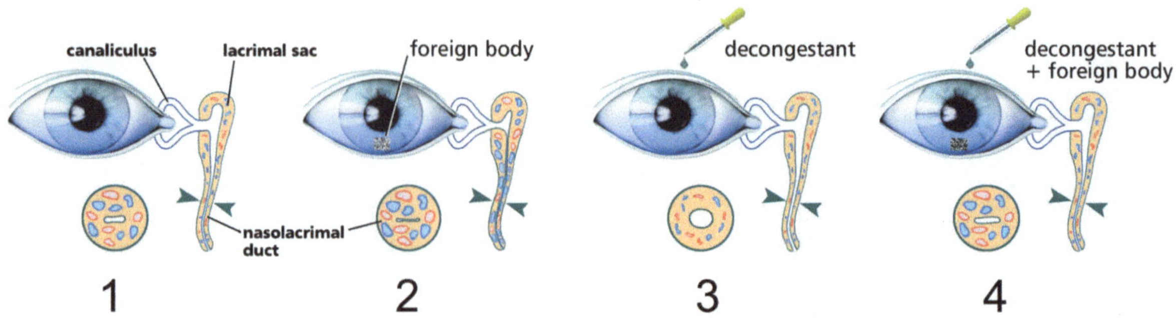

Fig. 1.10. Schematic/anatomical model of the state of the cavernous body and lacrimal passage in the resting state (*1*) and under different experimental conditions (*2–4*) indicating the specific swelling and compression of the cavernous body and how it permits or restricts tear drainage. (From [19])

are worn or not, or whether the person is suffering from a common cold or not [2].

1.3.4 Absorption of Tear-Fluid Components

Recent animal experiments have indicated that components of tear fluid are absorbed in the nasolacrimal passage and are transported into the surrounding cavernous body that is subject to autonomic control and regulates tear outflow (Table 1.2) [13]. Under normal conditions tear fluid components are constantly absorbed into the blood vessels of the surrounding cavernous body. These vessels are connected to the blood vessels of the outer eye and could act as a feedback signal for tear fluid production (Fig. 1.11) [13, 19], which ceases if these tear components are not absorbed (see Chap. 2).

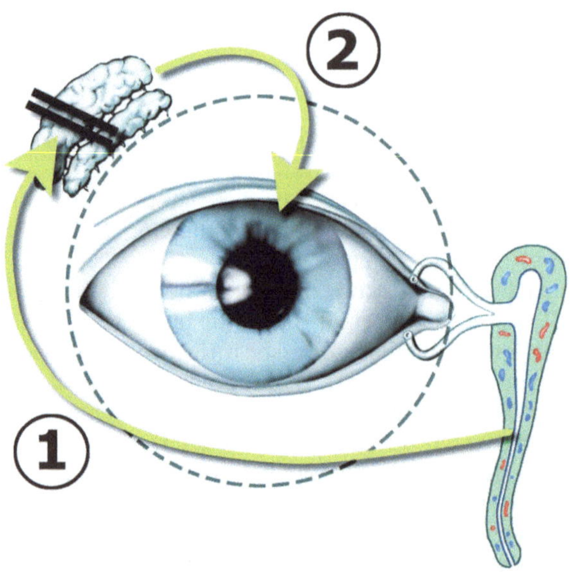

Fig. 1.11. The normally constant absorption of tear fluid components into the blood vessels of the surrounding cavernous body of the nasolacrimal ducts and their transport to the lacrimal gland by blood vessel connections (*1*) could be a feedback signal for tear fluid production (*2*). (From [19])

1.4 Conclusions

The human efferent tear ducts are part of the lacrimal system. They consist of the upper and the lower lacrimal canaliculus, the lacrimal sac, and the nasolacrimal duct. As a draining and secretory system, the nasolacrimal ducts play a decisive role in tear transport and nonspecific immune defense. In this context the integrity of the mucosa as source of mucins and trefoil factor family peptides is of great importance with regard to tear drainage. Moreover, components of tear fluid are absorbed by the epithelium of the nasolacrimal passage and are transported into a surrounding vascular system. This system is comparable to a cavernous body that is subject to autonomic control and regulates tear outflow. Tear duct-associated lymphoid tissue (TALT) is present in the efferent tear ducts, displaying the cytomorphological and immunophenotypic features of mucosa-associated lymphoid tissue (MALT).

Acknowledgements

I thank B. Tillmann for permitting to use Fig. 1.1 from his Atlas of Anatomy, C. Franke for providing schematic drawings (Figs. 1.3, 1.10, 1.11), and E. Axmann for editing the English. I thank Deutsche Forschungsgemeinschaft (PA 738/1-5) and Wilhelm-Roux program (grant FKZ 9/18) for support.

References

1. Akiyama J, Hoffman A, Brown C, Allen L, Edmondson J, Poulain F, Hawgood S (2002) Tissue distribution of surfactant proteins A and D in the mouse. J Histochem Cytochem 50:993–996
2. Ayub M, Thale A, Hedderich J, Tillmann B, Paulsen F (2003) The cavernous body of the human efferent tear ducts functions in regulation of tear outflow. Invest Ophthalmol Vis Sci 44:4900–4907
3. Belmonte C, Aracil A, Acosta C, Luna C, Gallar J (2004) Nerves and sensations from the eye surface. Ocular Surface 2:248–253
4. Gipson IK, Hori Y, Argüeso P (2004) Character of ocular surface mucins and their alteration in dry eye disease. Ocular Surface 2:131–148
5. Hoffmann W, Jagla W (2002) Cell type specific expression of secretory TFF peptides: colocalization with mucins and synthesis in the brain. Int Rev Cytol 213:147–181
6. Langer G, Jagla W, Behrens-Baumann W, Walter S, Hoffmann W (1999) Secretory peptides TFF1 and TFF3 synthesized in human conjunctival goblet cells. Invest Ophthalmol Vis Sci 40:2220–2224
7. McCulley JP, Shine WE (2003) Meibomian gland function and the tear lipid layer. Ocular Surface 1:97–106
8. McDermott (2004) Defensins and other antimicrobial peptides at the ocular surface. Ocular Surface 2:229–247
9. Paulsen F (2003) The nasolacrimal ducts. Adv Anat Embryol Cell Biol 170:1–106
10. Paulsen F, Berry M (2006) Mucins and TFF peptides of the tear film and lacrimal apparatus. Progr Histochem Cytochem 41:1–56
11. Paulsen F, Corfield A, Hinz M, Hoffmann W, Schaudig U, Thale A, Berry M (2003) Characterization of mucins in human lacrimal sac and nasolacrimal duct. Invest Ophthalmol Vis Sci 44:1807–1813
12. Paulsen F, Corfield A, Hinz M, Hoffmann W, Schaudig U, Thale A, Berry M (2004) Tränenabfluss – Bedeutung von Muzinen und TFF-Peptiden. Ophthalmologe 101:19–24
13. Paulsen F, Föge M, Thale A, Tillmann B, Mentlein R (2002) Absorption of lipophilic substances from tear fluid by the epithelium of the nasolacrimal ducts. Invest Ophthalmol Vis Sci 43:3137–3143
14. Paulsen F, Hallmann U, Paulsen J, Thale A (2000) Innervation of the cavernous body of the human efferent tear ducts and function in tear outflow mechanism. J Anat 197:373–381
15. Paulsen F, Hinz M, Schaudig U, Thale AB, Hoffmann W (2002) TFF-peptides in the human efferent tear ducts. Invest Ophthalmol Vis Sci 43:3359–3364
16. Paulsen F, Langer G, Hoffmann W, Berry M (2004) Human lacrimal gland mucins. Cell Tissue Res 316:167–177
17. Paulsen F, Paulsen J, Thale A, Tillmann B (2000) Mucosa-associated lymphoid tissue (MALT) in the human efferent tear ducts. Virchows Arch 437:185–189
18. Paulsen F, Pufe T, Schaudig U, Held-Feindt J, Lehmann J, Schröder J-M, Tillmann B (2001) Detection of natural peptide antibiotics in human nasolacrimal ducts. Invest Ophthalmol Vis Sci 42:2157–2163
19. Paulsen F, Schaudig U, Thale A (2003) Drainage of tears: impact on the ocular surface and lacrimal system. Ocular Surface 1:180–191
20. Paulsen F, Thale A, Hallmann U, Schaudig U, Tillmann B (2000) The cavernous body of the human efferent tear ducts: function in tear outflow mechanism. Invest Ophthalmol Vis Sci 41:965–970
21. Paulsen F, Thale A, Kohla G, Schauer R, Rochels R, Parwaresch R, Tillmann B (1998) Functional anatomy of human duct epithelium. Anat Embryol 198:1–12
22. Stern ME, Beuermann RW, Fox RI, Gao J, Mircheff AK, Pflugfelder SC (1998) The pathology of dry eye: the interaction between the ocular surface and lacrimal glands. Cornea 17:584–589
23. Stoeckelhuber M, Stoeckelhuber BM, Welsch U (2003) Human glands of Moll: histochemical and ultrastructural characterization of the glands of Moll in the human eyelid. J Invest Dermatol 121:28–36
24. Sullivan DA, Sullivan BD, Ullman MD, Rocha EM, Krenzer KL, Cermak JM, Toda I, Doane MG, Evans JE, Wickham LA (2000) Androgen influence on the Meibomian gland. Invest Ophthalmol Vis Sci 41:3732–3742
25. Thale A, Paulsen F, Rochels R, Tillmann B (1998) Functional anatomy of human efferent tear ducts: a new theory of tear outflow. Graefe's Arch Clin Exp Ophthalmol 236:674–678
26. Tillmann B (2005) Atlas der Anatomie. Springer, Berlin Heidelberg, New York
27. Lüllmann Rauch R (2003) Histologie. Thieme, Stuttgart

Chapter 2

Pathophysiological Aspects of PANDO, Dacryolithiasis, Dry Eye, and Punctum Plugs

2

Friedrich Paulsen

Core Messages

- Early cases of dacryostenosis are based on descending inflammation from the eye or ascending inflammation from the nose initiating swelling of the mucous membrane and malfunctions in the subepithelial cavernous body with reactive hyperemia, and temporary occlusion of the lacrimal passage.
- Repeated isolated occurrence of dacryocystitis leads to structural epithelial changes with loss of mucin and TFF peptide producing goblet cells and columnar epithelial cells, remodeling of the helical arrangement of subepithelial connective tissue fibers, and loss of specialized blood vessels of the subepithelial cavernous body.
- Structural epithelial and subepithelial changes lead either to a total fibrous closure of the lumen of the efferent tear duct or to a non-functional segment in the lacrimal passage that manifests on syringing.
- The first step in dacryolith formation seems to be a change in tear fluid rheology with the formation of a still only partly characterized amorphous material.
- In most cases, the material formed initiates an epithelial reaction with increased production of secretory components in the nasolacrimal passage, based perhaps on mechanical irritation or bacterial colonization with immigration of granulocytes and production of antimicrobial substances.
- Dacryoliths consist partly of secreted mucins that are comparable with the mucin spectrum of the epithelium of the healthy nasolacrimal ducts.
- Besides mucins, TFF peptides are augmented in dacryoliths and may have a functional role in dacryolith formation.
- It remains unknown whether TFF peptides per se influence dacryolith formation or whether their secretion as well as the secretion of mucins and defense substances is only a secondary phenomenon.
- Under normal conditions, tear-fluid components are constantly absorbed into the blood vessels of the surrounding cavernous body. These vessels are connected to the blood vessels of the outer eye and could act as a feedback signal for tear-fluid production, which ceases if these tear components are not absorbed. In this way, dry eye could be initiated.
- Punctum plugs could initially function by totally preventing absorption of tear-fluid components, thus creating an "empty" tear-fluid system, which may be a strong stimulation signal for tear-fluid production. This stimulation signal decreases over time. This may explain why nearly all patients after insertion of punctum plugs and other blocking methods – viewed in the long run – require tear substitutes.

- TALT may favor the rise of primary low-grade B-cell lymphoma of the MALT type.
- Analysis of TALT, as well as different epithelial cells of the lacrimal passage, are interesting with regard to the induction of tolerance in the nasolacrimal ducts and at the ocular surface.

Contents

2.1 Introduction

Dacryocystitis, dacryostenosis, and dacryolithiasis are the three major alterations of the human nasolacrimal ducts the clinican is confronted with in his/her daily practice. Hardly any malignancies occur in the efferent tear-duct system. The leading symptom of most patients is epiphora. The present chapter summarizes recent advances in the understanding of the pathophysiology of dacryostenosis and dacryolithiasis. Moreover, it also discusses current considerations regarding the involvement of the nasolacrimal ducts with dry eye and the benefit of uncoupling the efferent tear-duct system from the ocular surface by punctum plugs.

2.2 Primary Aquired Nasolacrimal Duct Obstruction

Idiopathic or primary acquired daryostenosis, synonymous with primary acquired nasolacrimal duct obstruction (PANDO), is a syndrome of unknown origin. Of all non-traumatic forms, it accounts for most cases observed in adults. Pathological studies of the nasolacrimal passage have indicated that PANDO is caused by fibrous obstruction secondary to chronic inflammation [4, 13, 14]. Nevertheless, the pathophysiology of functional dacryostenosis, i.e., patients with epiphora despite patent lacrimal passages on syringing (so-called functional dacryostenosis) has still not been understood. Descending pathogens from the conjunctival sac, as well as diverticula of the lacrimal passage, have been suggested to be causal factors. Other specialists claim to have located the origin of idiopathic dacryostenosis in the nose. Here, simple infections of the nasal mucous membrane or diseases of the sinuses have been suggested; however, clinical studies indicate that nasal disease is extremely rare in patients undergoing dacryocystorhinostomy (DCR).

Interestingly, the mucous membranes of the lacrimal passage and nose reveal morphological differences between the nasolacrimal epithelial cells with microciliation only and the nasal epithelial cells with their kinociliae (Fig. 2.1) [24]. This suggests differences in susceptibility to pathogens; however, it has been shown that ectopia of nasal epithelial cells is a more or less common finding in the nasolacrimal ducts [1, 27]. In addition to descending infection from the eye, ascending infection of these atopical cells during nasal inflammation could thus be the starting point of dacryostenosis. In this scenario, the nasal inflammation has long since abated when the dacryocystitis passes into a chronic state, causing the changes characteristic for dacryostenosis (see below).

Recent findings have indicated that "functional obstruction" of the lacrimal passage occurs in many more patients than suggested previously (Table 2.1) [25]. Furthermore, some of these patients report a history of acute or chronic dacryocystitis and digital pressure over the sac also reveals mucopurulent reflux in some cases [25].

Squamous metaplasia has been observed during recent analyses in cases of functional dacryostenosis with loss of columnar epithelial cells and goblet cells and with that of lacrimal passage specific mucins and TFF peptides (see Chap. 1) in the stenotic area (Figs. 2.2, 2.3). Moreover, the helically arranged connective tissue fibers undergo remodeling leading to subepithelial fibrosis (Fig. 2.2) [25]. In addition, a reduction and even total loss of specialized blood vessels of the surrounding cavernous body and their replacement by connective tissue occurs (Fig. 2.2) [25].

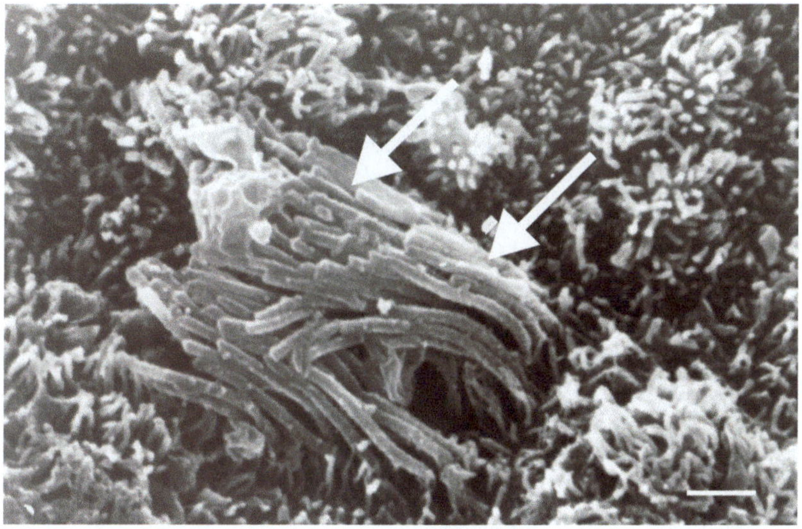

Fig. 2.1. Scanning electron micrograph of the epithelial surface of the nasolacrimal duct reveals a single cell with kinociliae (*arrows*) between cells with microvilli. Bar=6 µm

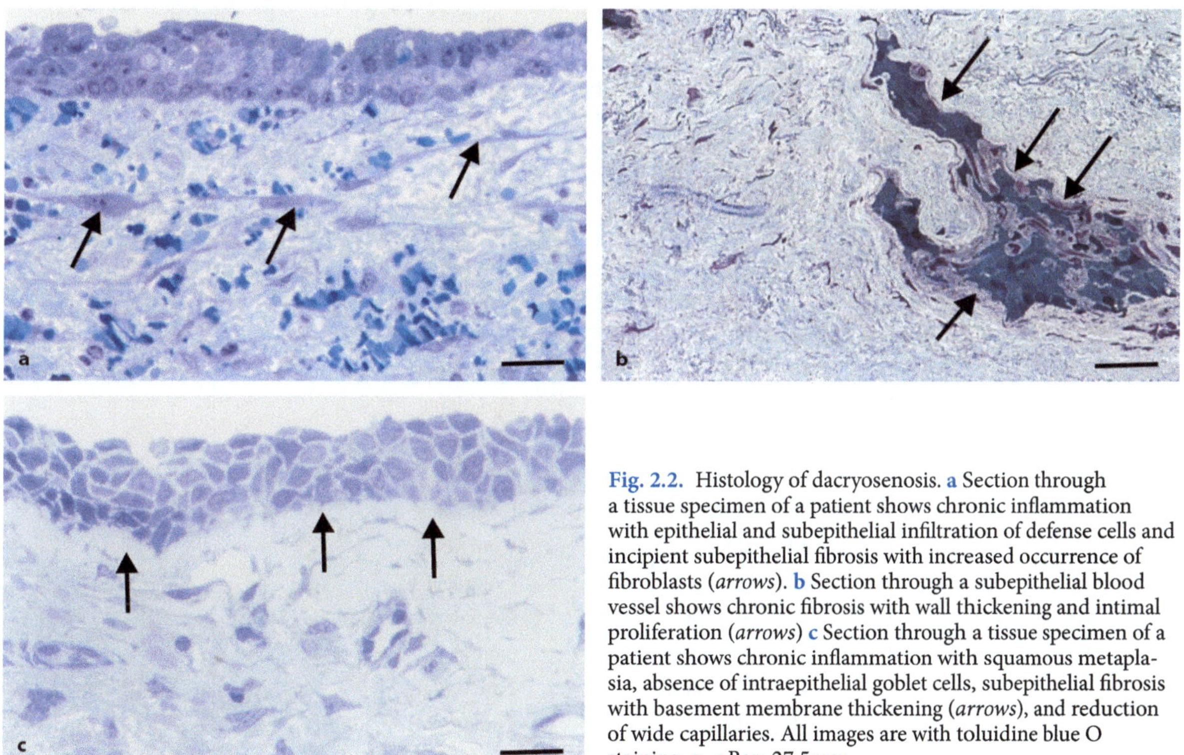

Fig. 2.2. Histology of dacryosenosis. **a** Section through a tissue specimen of a patient shows chronic inflammation with epithelial and subepithelial infiltration of defense cells and incipient subepithelial fibrosis with increased occurrence of fibroblasts (*arrows*). **b** Section through a subepithelial blood vessel shows chronic fibrosis with wall thickening and intimal proliferation (*arrows*) **c** Section through a tissue specimen of a patient shows chronic inflammation with squamous metaplasia, absence of intraepithelial goblet cells, subepithelial fibrosis with basement membrane thickening (*arrows*), and reduction of wide capillaries. All images are with toluidine blue O staining. **a–c** Bar=27.5 µm

Table 2.1. Patient case data of a group of 36 patients undergoing endonasal dacryocystorhinostomy in PANDO at the Department of Otorhinolaryngology, Head and Neck Surgery, Christian Albrecht University of Kiel, Germany. *DE* duration of epiphora (months), *LS* lacrimal sac, *ND* nasolacrimal duct, *DC* dacryocystitis, *MD* mucous discharge. (From [25])

Case no.	Gender	Age (years)	Side	DE	Patho-logical stage	Stenosis location	Degree of obstruction	DC	MD	Sinusitis or nasal disease
1	F	64	L	21	Severe	LS	Functional	X		
2	F	50	R	120	Severe	LS/ND	Complete	X	X	
3	M	92	L	12	Severe	ND	Complete			Acute sinusitis
4	F	32	L	6	Mild	ND	Functional			
5	F	75	L	157	Severe	ND	Complete	X	X	
6	F	48	L	26	Moderate	ND	Functional	X		
7	F	69	R	8	Moderate	LS/ND	Complete	X	X	
8	F	73	R	27	Severe	LS/ND	Complete	X	X	
9	F	39	R	19	Severe	ND	Complete			
10	F	57	L	9	Moderate	ND	Complete			
11	F	40	R	13	Moderate	LS/ND	Functional			
12	F	45	R	36	Severe	ND	Complete	X	X	
13	F	67	L	204	Severe	ND	Functional	X	X	Chronic sinusitis
14	F	63	R	4	Mild	LS/ND	Functional			
15	F	58	L	13	Moderate	LS/ND	Complete	X	X	
16	M	76	R	27	Severe	LS	Complete	X	X	
17	F	16	L	20	Moderate	ND	Complete			
18	F	41	R	7	Mild	LS	Functional	X		
19	M	32	R	15	Moderate	LS	Complete			
20	M	55	R	24	Severe	ND	Complete	X	X	
21	F	60	R	120	Severe	ND	Functional	X		
22	F	66	L	240	Severe	LS	Functional	X	X	
23	F	28	L	7	Mild	ND	Functional			
24	F	61	R	240	Severe	ND	Functional	X		
25	M	36	R	49	Severe	LS/ND	Complete	X	X	
26	F	55	L	16	Severe	LS/ND	Complete	X	X	Nasal sinusitis
27	M	65	L	14	Moderate	ND	Complete			
28	F	79	L	36	Severe	ND	Complete			
29	F	21	L	20	Severe	LS	Complete	X	X	
30	F	88	R	1	Moderate	ND	Complete			
31	F	61	L	12	Moderate	ND	Functional			Nasal sinusitis
32	F	60	L	10	Mild	LS	Functional			
33	F	51	R	32	Severe	ND	Complete	X	X	
34	F	45	L	49	Severe	LS/ND	Complete	X	X	
35	F	70	L	29	Severe	ND	Complete			
36	F	61	L	59	Severe	LS/ND	Complete			

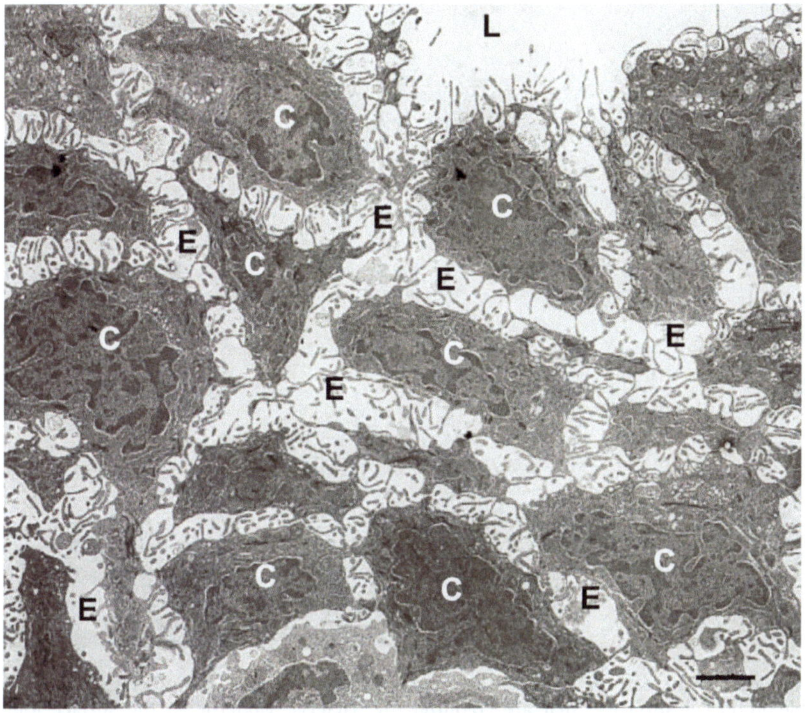

Fig. 2.3. Transmission electron micrograph reveals chronic stage of dacryostenosis. The epithelium shows squamous metaplasia. The metaplastic squamous cells reveal condensed, irregular nuclei (*C*), reduction of cytoplasm, and reduction of cell organelles. The cell surface shows a loose microciliation projecting into a large extracellular space (*E*). *L* lumen of the lacrimal passage. Bar=6 µm

All these changes lead to an interruption of the tear-flow mechanism in the stenotic segment. The following pathogenic concept of primary acquired dacryostenosis has been postulated: descending inflammation from the eye or ascending inflammation from the region of the nose (perhaps by way of inflammation of "ectopical" nasal epithelial cells in the nasolacrimal duct; Fig. 2.4) may initiate malfunctions in the cavernous body with reactive hyperemia, swelling of the mucous membrane, and temporary occlusion of the lacrimal passage [25]. Then, repeated isolated episodes of dacryocystitis may lead to structural epithelial and subepithelial changes. Loss of typical goblet and epithelial cells, which plays an important role in the tear-outflow mechanism, as well as fibrosis of the helical system of connective tissue fibers in the area of the lacrimal sac and nasolacrimal duct and reduction and destruction of specialized blood vessels of the cavernous body, may exacerbate malfunctions of the tear-outflow mechanism and start a vicious circle [25]; thus, cases of functional dacryostenosis, i.e., patients with epiphora in spite of patent lacrimal passages on syringing, are explainable as follows:

1. In early cases, the rinsing liquid instilled by hand pressure into the lacrimal passage is forced through the segment of the lacrimal passage obturated by reactive hyperemia and swelling of the mucous membrane.
2. Structural changes (caused by chronic dacryocystitis) result in a non-functioning segment in the lacrimal passage. In this latter case, obstruction is not yet complete, but there is no tear transport in the non-functioning segment [25].

Ample evidence certainly exists that obstructed nasolacrimal systems are colonized by increased numbers of pathogenic microorganisms. The histopathology implies that, besides topical or systemic anti-inflammatory agents, nasal decongestants, such as Afrin, possibly could also be useful tools in the management of early cases of primary acquired dacryostenosis, since they could counteract the hyperemia and swelling of the cavernous body [25].

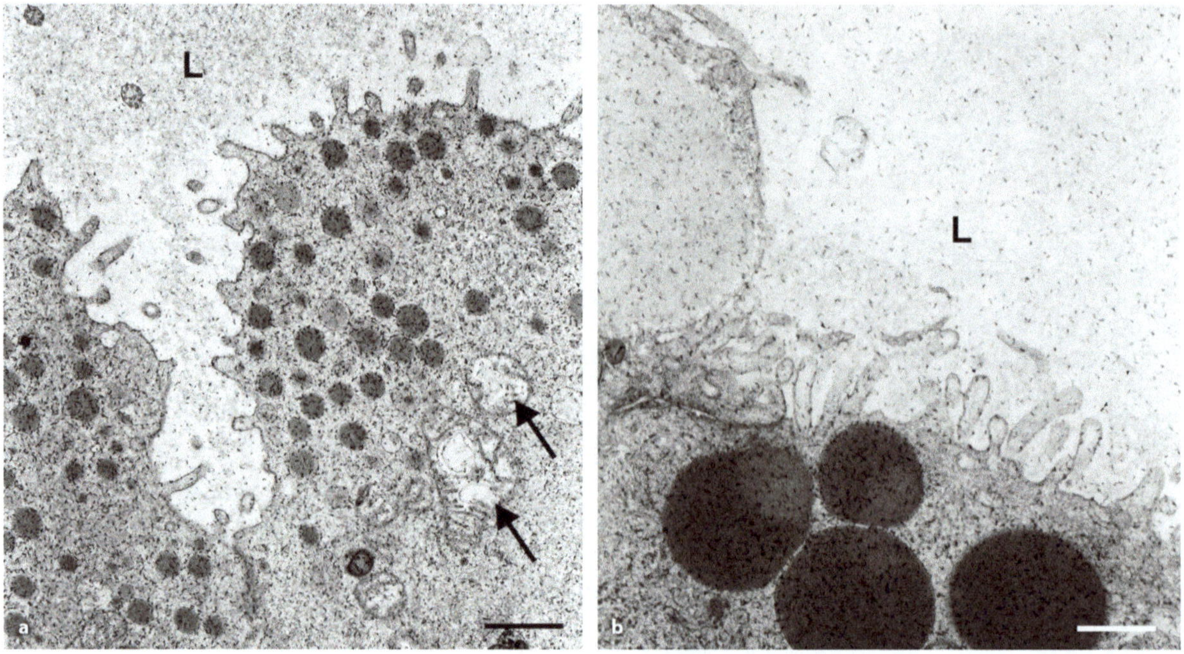

Fig. 2.4. Transmission electron micrograph reveals an early stage of dacryostenosis. **a** Bacteria are visible on the cell surface of two epithelial cells and in their cytoplasm infiltrating the cell organelles. Mitochondria indicated by *arrows*. **b** High magnification of the surface of an epithelial cell demonstrates microvilli that are colonized by bacteria. Underneath the surface four fat vacuoles are visible. *L* lumen of the lacrimal passage. **a** Bar=1.2 μm; **b** bar=0.4 μm

2.3 Dacryolithiasis

Dacryoliths (lacrimal stones) or "calculi" of the nasolacrimal ducts (Fig. 2.5) were described by Cesoni in as early as 1670 [12], and have been reported to occur in between 6 and 18% of patients with nasolacrimal duct obstruction who undergo dacryocystorhinostomy (DCR). They are one of the causes of PANDO. Dacryoliths may occur in any part of the nasolacrimal system, albeit most commonly in the lacrimal sac. Several predisposing factors have been suggested, such as increased occurrence in females, patient age below 50 years, association with cigarette smoking and facial-sinonasal trauma, and increased frequency subsequent to previous occurrence of dacryocystitis. However, other studies have indicated increased frequency in males and patients aged above 50 years; therefore, it seems that both genders are involved to nearly the same extent. Dacryoliths usually become symptomatic when they obstruct the nasolacrimal system. This can result in epiphora, acute dacryocystitis, protrusion of the lacrimal canthal region, and partial closure of the lacrimal passage (recognized during syringing by the ophthalmologist). Interestingly, dacryoliths occur more often in patients with partial and incomplete closure of the lacrimal passage (i.e., patients with epiphora despite patent lacrimal passages on syringing).

Scanning electron microscopy has shown that dacryoliths are composed of lobes and lobules built on an amorphous core material (Fig. 2.6; Table 2.2) [18]. Atomic absorption spectrophotometric investigations demonstrate that dacryoliths consist almost entirely of organic proteins and, to a much lesser extent, of inorganic material [18]. According to Lew et al. [11], lacrimal fluid from patients with dacryoliths contains a reduced amount of lysozyme and a lower calcium concentration than normal lacrimal fluid (Table 2.2). It is important to recognize that daryoliths are not calcified or are composed of any other "hard" substances (Table 2.2). Some stones reveal hyphae-like structures, although no fungi were recovered by culturing (Table 2.2) [18].

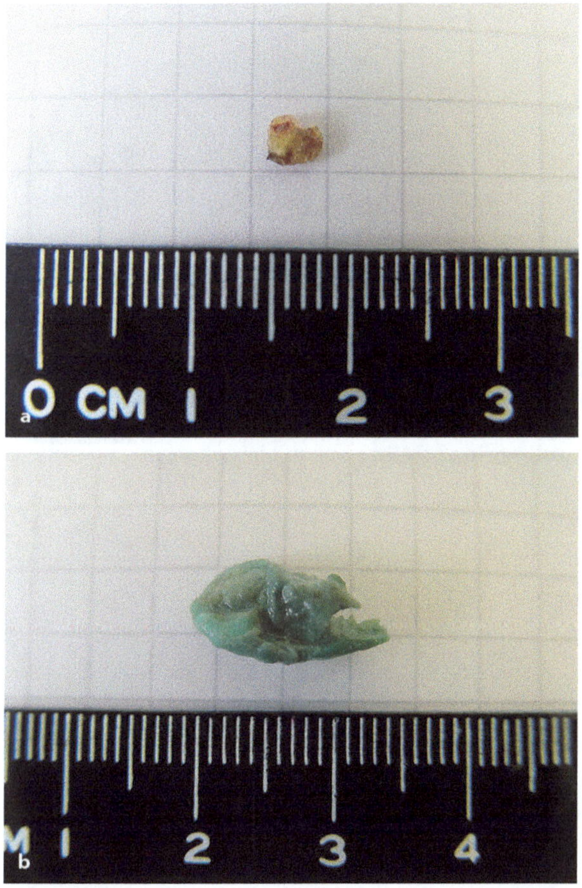

Fig. 2.5. Lacrimal sac dacryoliths immediately after dacryocystorhinostomy. a Dacryolith from a 61-year-old man. b Dacryolith of a 64-year-old woman

Table 2.2. Composition of dacryoliths

Lobes and lobules built on an amorphous core material
Almost entirely organic proteins
Nearly no inorganic material; not calcified; no "hard" substances
Reduced amounts of lysozyme and low calcium concentration in tear fluid from patients with dacryoliths
Some dacryoliths reveal hyphae-like structures
Parts of the amorphous core proteins stain with alcian blue (pH 1)
Parts of the amorphous core proteins contain mucins, especially MUC8 seems to be augmented
Parts of the amophous core proteins contain TFF peptides; TFF2 is induced in dacryoliths; TFF1 and TFF3 are augmented
Few cells are found in the amorphous core material of dacryoliths; these are mainly granulocytes and shredded epithelial cells and single T- and B-lymphocytes as well as macrophages

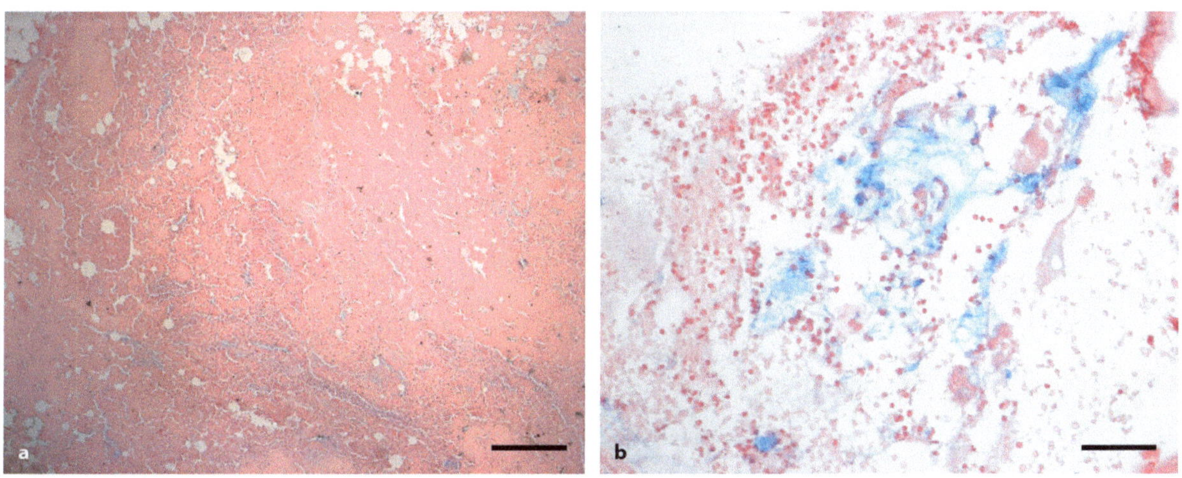

Fig. 2.6. Microscopic appearance of dacryoliths. a Lacrimal sac dacryolith reveals scant cellular material and amorphous debris. Hematoxylin–eosin staining. b Part of a dacryolith with scant cellular material as well as a little amorphous material staining with alcian blue (pH 2.5) blue. a, b Bar=27.5 μm

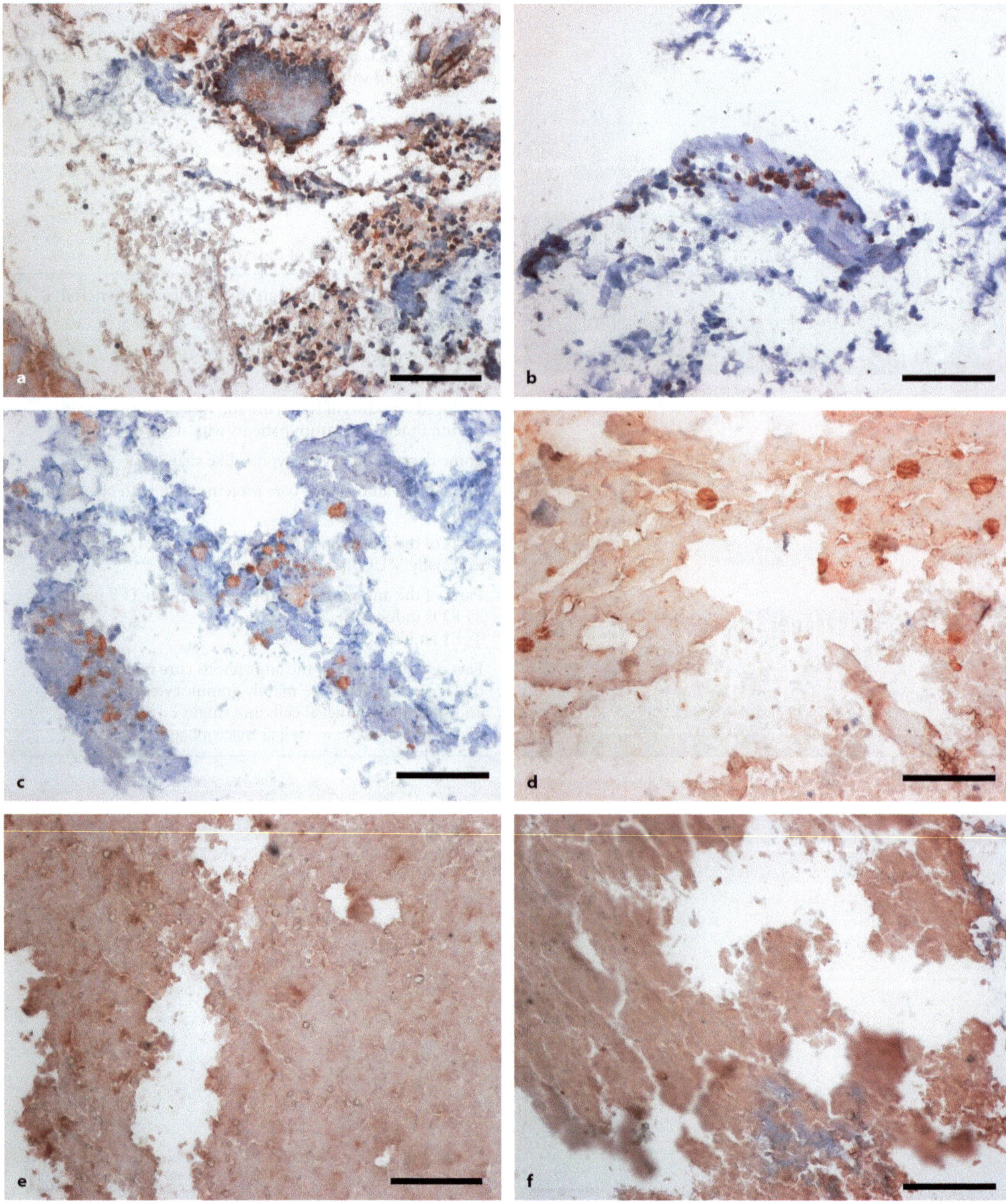

Fig. 2.7. Immunohistochemical detection of neutrophils (a), B-lymphocytes (b), mucin MUC2 (c), TFF1 (d), TFF2 (e), and TFF3 (f). a–f Bar=73 µm

Recent findings have indicated that parts of the amorphous core proteins stain with PAS and alcian blue (Fig. 2.6) and react with antibodies to mucins and TFF peptides (Fig. 2.7) [20]. Moreover, these findings show that most dacryoliths contain single cells and cellular debris. Most of these cells seem to be neutrophils that produce alpha defensins 1–3. Also, the calcium-dependent enzyme secretory phospholipase A_2 is present in many dacryoliths, indicating a host defense reaction against Gram-positive pathogens. A few T and B lymphocytes and macrophages have been detected, too (Table 2.2). It was demonstrated that a changed production of mucins and TFF peptides occurs in dacryoliths [20]. Mucins and TFF peptides are distributed as smaller or larger conglomerations in dacryoliths [20]. This distribution pattern is mostly in conformity with the mucin and TFF peptide repertoire of the healthy epithelium of the lacrimal sac and nasolacrimal duct. Production of MUC1, 2, 4, 5AC and 5B was observed in most dacryoliths, but not all, whereas reactivity for MUC3, 6, and 7 was only detected in a few cases. Interestingly, MUC8 was visible in nearly all investigated dacryoliths and revealed strong staining intensity [20].

The most interesting finding in dacryolithiasis, however, was the strong staining of TFF peptides in dacryoliths, suggesting upregulation of TFF peptides in dacryolithiasis [32]. RT-PCR and immunohistochemistry revealed expression and production of all three TFF peptides, whereas in the healthy situation only TFF1 and TFF3 are expressed and produced, indicating that induction of TFF2 occurs in dacryolithiasis. Analysis by real-time PCR revealed increased expression levels of TFF1 and TFF3 [20]; thus, TFF2 seems to be induced in dacryolithiasis, whereas TFF1 and TFF3 are augmented (Table 2.2). A comparable finding has just recently been published in the biliary tract where it was shown that all three TFF peptides are augmented in hepatolithiasis.

The increased TFF peptides may play a role in dacryolithogenesis together with oversecreted mucins. The TFFs alter the physiological properties of the secreted mucin, leading to an increase in the optical density and viscosity of purified mucin preparations when added in vitro. TFF1 interacting proteins are MUC2 and MUC5AC. The binding regions are VWFC1 and VWFC2 cysteine-rich domains, possibly raising the viscosity of the mucin. It has also been suggested that TFF2 and TFF3 may act as link peptides and thereby influence the rheological properties of mucous gels. Given the increased production of TFFs in dacryolithiasis, it is likely that TFFs may couple with MUC5AC and MUC2, and possibly with other mucins (MUC8) as well, and contribute to increased tear-film viscosity of the mucins drained through the nasolacrimal passage [8, 31].

The first step in dacryolith formation could be a change in tear-fluid rheology with the formation of a yet uncharacterized amorphous material (hypothetically the amorphous material might consist of degraded substances of the ocular tear-film components and develops based on water extraction by the epithelium of the nasolacrimal ducts from causes as yet unknown). In most cases, the material formed initiates an epithelial reaction with increased production of secretory components (TFF peptides, distinct mucins) in the nasolacrimal passage, based perhaps on mechanical irritation or bacterial colonization with immigration of granulocytes and production of antimicrobial substances. Fungal colonization also seems to occur in some cases. In this scenario, differences in the composition of dacryoliths with regard to mucins and defense cells may be explained by colonization with distinct bacteria; however, it is not clear yet whether dacryolith formation occurs as a reaction to previous inflammation of the nasolacrimal ducts or whether other factors, such as drugs (perhaps different eye drops), changes in the hormonal status, or immunmodulation (allergy), may lead to the initiation of dacryolith formation with recurrent dacryocystitis as a secondary phenomenon.

Finally, the question remains whether TFF peptides and mucins per se influence dacryolith formation, or whether their secretion is only a secondary phenomenon. A full understanding of the molecular function of TFF peptides and mucins at the mucosal surface of the efferent tear duct passage will provide further insight into the occurrence of dacryolithiasis, which often leads to residual functional impairment with epiphora.

2.4 Dry Eye and Punctum Plugs: Impact of Tear Drainage

The Dry Eye Workshop 2004, at the Puerto Rico TFOS (Tear Film and Ocular Surface Society) conference, defined dry eye (also termed sicca syndrome or keratoconjunctivitis sicca) as a multi-factorial disorder of tears and the ocular surface, associated with

Table 2.3. Summary of dry eye disease

Multifactorial disorder of tears and the ocular surface
Associated with symptoms of discomfort and/or visual disturbance
Pathological features include increased epithelial stratification and proliferative index and abnormal differentiation with maintenance of a basal phenotype
Reduced expression of secretory and membrane-bound mucins by the superficial ocular-surface epithelial cells
Worsened severity as aqueous tear secretion decreases and as the ability to reflex tears in response to sensory stimulation is lost
Disease results in a vicious cycle
The normally constant absorption of tear-fluid components into the blood vessels of the surrounding cavernous body could come to halt if these tear components are not absorbed, and thus could initiate dry eye

symptoms of discomfort and/or visual disturbance (Table 2.3). Much is known about the pathogenesis of the keratoconjunctivitis sicca that occurs in dry eye disease (Table 2.3). The pathological features of this condition include increased epithelial stratification and proliferative index and abnormal differentiation with maintenance of a basal phenotype (Table 2.3) [9]. Furthermore, the expression of secretory and membrane-bound mucins by the superficial ocular surface epithelial cells is reduced (Table 2.3) [3, 6, 26]. An exact mechanism for the development of these pathological changes has not yet been elucidated. The severity of keratoconjunctivitis sicca worsens as aqueous tear secretion decreases and as the ability to reflex tear in response to sensory stimulation is lost. The disease results in a vicious cycle.

Clinical reports have suggested that tear production and outflow of tears from the ocular surface are linked [16, 17]. As described in Chap. 1, the human nasolacrimal ducts have absorptive functions. Based on this, hypothetically it could be suggested that the normally constant absorption of tear-fluid components into the blood vessels of the surrounding cavernous body, which are connected to the blood vessels of the ocular surface, could provide a signal for tear-fluid production, which ceases when these tear components are not absorbed [23].

If this hypothesis is true, the question remains: Why do not all possible forms of efferent tear-duct diseases that are related to tear-outflow disturbances lead to dry eye? And why do punctum plugs and other methods that interrupt the connection between the ocular surface and the nasolacrimal ducts sometimes show very good results in the therapy of dry eye? These questions can be answered as follows:

1. Currently, little is known about whether diseases of the drainage system coincide with changes in tear-fluid production, although patients with diseases of the nasolacrimal ducts suffer from tear overflow. On the other hand, it has been reported that patients with acquired obstruction of the efferent tear ducts rarely have symptoms of epiphora [5, 7], and lack of significant epiphora has also been reported in patients with congenital absence of lacrimal puncta [2]. Moreover, as already mentioned, there are patients who suffer from functional dacryostenosis, i.e., patients with epiphora in spite of patent lacrimal passages on syringing.
2. Both dry eye and diseases of the efferent tear ducts occur with high frequency in women of middle to advanced age [15].
3. Considering the results after insertion of punctum plugs and other blocking methods, one can ascertain that patients, in the long run, require tear substitutes. Punctum plugs could initially function by totally preventing absorption of tear-fluid components, thus creating an "empty" tear-fluid system, which may be a strong stimulation signal for tear-fluid production. This stimulation signal decreases with passing of time. Ocular surface sensation and tear production also decrease after temporary punctual occlusion in normal subjects [30]. These effects are more pronounced in subjects with both upper and lower puncta occluded; however, in normal subjects, there appears to be an autoregulatory mechanism that returns tear production and tear clearance to preocclusion levels 14–17 days after punctual occlusion, a mechanism that seems to be lacking in dry-eye patients [30].

The apparently contradictory findings raised above under point 1 above can be explained as follows: Cases of acquired obstruction of the lacrimal drainage system or congenital absence of lacrimal puncta result from fibrous obstruction secondary to chronic

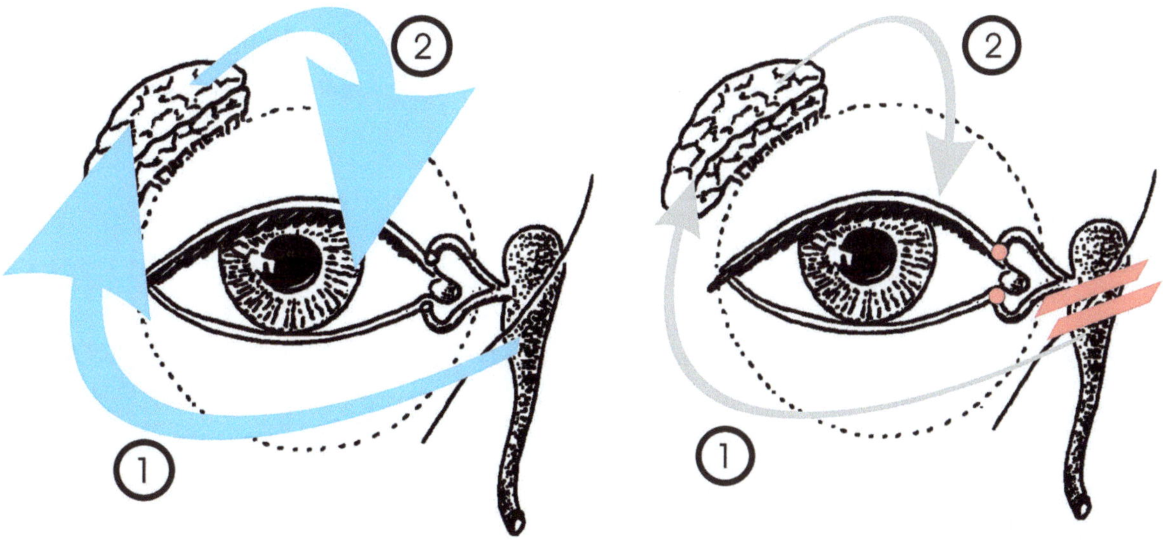

Fig. 2.8. The normally constant absorption of tear-fluid components into the blood vessels of the surrounding cavernous body of the nasolacrimal ducts and their transport to the lacrimal gland by blood vessel connections (*1*) could be a feedback signal for tear-fluid production (*2; left*) that comes to a halt if the nasolacrimal system has been occluded by punctum plugs (right)

inflammation, with total obstruction of the whole lacrimal sac and nasolacrimal duct [4, 13, 14]. This scenario is comparable to the insertion of punctum plugs, as absorption of tear-fluid components is totally prevented and the production of tear fluid is downregulated by the lacrimal gland, leading to symptoms of epiphora (Fig. 2.8). In the second case (patients with epiphora in spite of patent lacrimal passages on syringing), a non-functioning segment in the lacrimal passage results from advanced structural changes with loss of specialized blood vessels of the cavernous body, with changes in the helical organization of connective tissue, and with epithelial metaplasia caused by chronic dacryocystitis (see section 2.2) [25]. In this latter case, obstruction is not yet complete, but no tear transport takes place in the non-functioning segment. In this scenario, there is absorption of tear-fluid components in the area lying in front of the non-functioning segment [25], leading to normal tear-fluid production; however, as tear fluid is not drained, or is only minimally drained, a tear overflow results.

Disturbances in one part of the "lacrimal functional unit" (see Chap. 1, section 1.2.4) can have effects on all participant structures. As greater knowledge is gained about the regulation of the lacrimal gland/ocular surface/efferent tear duct integrated unit, new paradigms may emerge regarding which patients with dry-eye disease may benefit from punctual occlusion and which patients may suffer consequences.

2.5 Primary Low-Grade B-Cell Lymphoma of the MALT Type and Immune Deviation

The occurrence of mucosa-associated lymphoid tissue (MALT) is not a ubiquitous finding in the nasolacrimal ducts (although it is a feature commonly found in symptomatically normal nasolacrimal ducts) [19] and is acquired in response to antigenic stimulation. Loss of tear-duct-associated lymphoid tissue (TALT) seems to be associated with the scarring of symptomatic dacryostenosis, suggesting that the presence per se of TALT does not lead to scarring [21]. Whether special types of bacteria, viruses, allergic reactions, or other factors, such as some type of immune deviation (see below), are responsible for the development of TALT in humans is not clear at present; however, the occurrence of TALT may favor the rise of primary low-grade B-cell lymphoma of the MALT

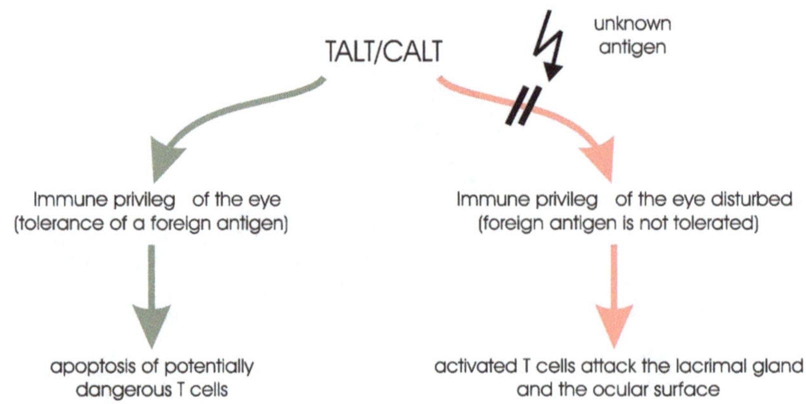

Fig. 2.9. Possible meaning of tear-duct (*TALT*) or conjunctiva (*CALT*) associated lymphoid tissue in the pathogenesis of dry eye

type, as has been shown by Kheterpal et al. [10], White et al. [29], and Tucker et al. [28].

Within the scope of this chapter it is impossible to review special immunological features of the eye; however, it should be mentioned that the anterior eye chamber (comparable to brain, placenta, testicle) has a special immunological state of reduced activation of the specific and non-specific immune system. This condition of local immune suppression, termed the immune privilege, is expressed in delayed or totally suppressed rejection of allogenic transplantations in these organs. This is illustrated in the survival of corneal and lens transplants in the anterior eye chamber and is called immune tolerance. It is known that such tolerance is transferable by injection into a second animal of splenocytes from an animal that was primed by inoculation of an antigen, demonstrating that antigens from the anterior eye chamber receive a signal that produces immune deviation and that regulatory T-cells have developed.

Recent analysis indicates that defective stimulation of TALT (Fig. 2.9) could result in abnormal immune deviation at the ocular surface leading to an autoimmunological response that causes dry-eye pathology. For more and detailed explanation see work by Paulsen et al. [22].

2.6 Conclusions

As described, the human nasolacrimal ducts must be included in the considerations concerning dry eye. Areas of interest include analyses of normal tear components, such as mucins, TFF peptides, and freely water-soluble small molecules (e.g., urea or amino acids), or perhaps smaller molecular tear proteins such as lysozyme. Moreover, analysis of such molecules in certain diseases, such as dacryostenosis, are of interest. Such investigations would be useful for extrapolation to the human situation, as the exact mechanism of absorption and regulation of these processes at the mucosa of the lacrimal passage is still not understood. Current investigations of epithelial transporter systems of the human nasolacrimal ducts will give deeper insights into possible routes of absorption and also the substances that are able to be absorbed. Possibly, some of these transporters are regulated by hormones in the efferent tear ducts, similar to the action of the water transporter aquaporine (AQP) 2 in the kidney, where AQP2 is only present in the apical membrane of collecting duct main cells under the influence of adiuretic hormone. Moreover, current analysis of TALT and also conjunctiva-associated lymphoid tissue (CALT), as well as different epithelial cells of the lacrimal passage, are interesting with regard to the induction of tolerance in the nasolacrimal system and at the ocular surface.

Acknowledgements

I thank E. Axmann for editing the English, and Deutsche Forschungsgemeinschaft PA 738/1-5 and Wilhelm-Roux program (grant FKZ 9/18) for support.

References

1. Adenis JP, Loubet A, Leboutet MJ, Robin A, Loubet R (1980) Morphologie ultrastructurale de la muqueuse des voies lacrymalesà ses différents niveaux. Arch Anat Cytol Pathol 28:371–375
2. Allen JC (1968) Congenital absence of the lacrimal punctum. J Pediatr Ophthalmol 5:176–178
3. Argüeso P, Balaram M, Spurr-Michaud S, Keutmann HT, Dana MR, Gipson IK (2002) Decreased levels of the goblet cell mucin MUC5AC in tears of patients with Sjögren syndrome. Invest Ophthalmol Vis Sci 43:1004–1011
4. Busse H, Müller KM (1977) Zur Entstehung der idiopathischen Dakryostenose. Klin Monatsbl Augenheilkd 170: 627–632
5. Dalgleish R (1964) Incidence of idiopathic acquired obstructions in the lacrimal drainage apparatus. Br J Ophthalmol 48:373–376
6. Danjo Y, Watanabe H, Tisdale AS, George M, Tsumura T, Abelson MB, Gipson IK (1998) Alterations of mucin in human conjunctival epithelia in dry eye. Invest Ophthalmol Vis Sci 39:2602–2609
7. François J, Neetens A (1973) Tear flow in man. Am J Ophthalmol 75:351–358
8. Paulsen F (2006) Cell and molecular biology of human lacrimal gland and nasolacrimal duct mucins. Int Rev Cytol 249:229–279
9. Jones DT, Ji A, Monroy D, Ji Z, Pflugfelder SC (1998) Alterations of ocular surface gene expression in Sjogren's syndrome. Adv Exp Med Biol 438:533–536
10. Kheterpal S, Chan SY, Batch A, Kirkby GR (1994) Previously undiagnosed lymphoma presenting as recurrent dacryocystitis. Arch Ophthalmol 112:519–520
11. Lew H, Lee S-Y, Yun Y-S (2004) Measurement of pH, electrolytes and electrophoretic studies of tear proteins in tears of patients with dacryoliths: a novel concept for dacryoliths. Ophthalmologica 218:130–135
12. Linberg JV (2001) Discussion of lacrimal sac dacryoliths. Ophthalmology 108:1312
13. Linberg JV, McCormick SA (1986) Primary acquired nasolacrimal duct obstruction. A clinical pathologic report and biopsy technique. Ophthalmology 93:1055–1063
14. Mauriello JA, Palydowycz S, DeLuca J (1992) Clinicopathologic study of lacrimal sac and nasal mucosa in 44 patients with complete acquired nasolacrimal duct obstruction. Ophthalmic Plast Reconstr Surg 8:13–21
15. McCarty CA, Bansal AK, Livingston PM, Stanislavsky YL, Taylor HR (1998) The epidemiology of dry eye in Melbourne, Australia. Ophthalmology 105:1114–1119
16. Mishima S (1965) Some physiological aspects of the precorneal tear film. Arch Ophthalmol 73:233–241
17. Norn MS (1966) Tear secretion in diseased eyes. Acta Ophthalmol 44:25–32
18. Orhan M, Onerci M, Dayanir V, Orhan D, Irkec T, Irkec M (1996) Lacrimal sac dacryolith: a study with atomic absorption spectrophotometry and scanning electron microscopy. Eur J Ophthalmol 6:478–480
19. Paulsen F, Paulsen J, Thale A, Tillmann B (2000) Mucosa-associated lymphoid tissue (MALT) in the human efferent tear ducts. Virchows Arch 437:185–189
20. Paulsen F, Schaudig U, Fabian A, Ehrich D, Sel S (in press) Production of TFF peptides and single mucins is augmented in dacryolithiasis. Graefe's Arch Clin Exp Ophthalmol
21. Paulsen F, Schaudig U, Maune S, Thale AB (2003) Loss of tear duct-associated lymphoid tissue (TALT) in association with the scarring of symptomatic dacryostenosis. Ophthalmology 110:85–92
22. Paulsen F, Schaudig U, Thale A (2003) Drainage of tears: impact on the ocular surface and lacrimal system. Ocular Surface 1:180–191
23. Paulsen F, Thale A, Hallmann U, Schaudig U, Tillmann B (2000) The cavernous body of the human efferent tear ducts: function in tear outflow mechanism. Invest Ophthalmol Vis Sci 41:965–970
24. Paulsen F, Thale A, Kohla G, Schauer R, Rochels R, Parwaresch R, Tillmann B (1998) Functional anatomy of human duct epithelium. Anat Embryol 198:1–12
25. Paulsen F, Thale A, Maune S, Tillmann B (2001) Primary acquired dacryostenosis: histopathology and pathophysiology. Ophthalmology 108:2329–2336
26. Pflugfelder SC, Tseng SC, Yoshino K, Monroy D, Felix C, Reis BL (1997) Correlation of goblet cell density and mucosal epithelial membrane mucin expression with rose bengal staining in patients with ocular irritations. Ophthalmology 104:223–235
27. Radnot M (1970) Die Flimmerhaare des Tränensackepithels. Klin Monatsbl Augenheilkd 170:428–432
28. Tucker N, Chow D, Stockl F, Codere F, Burnier M (1997) Clinically suspected primary acquired nasolacrimal duct obstruction. Ophthalmology 104:1882–1886
29. White WL, Ferry JA, Harris NL, Grove AS Jr (1995) Ocular adnexal lymphoma. Ophthalmology 102:1994–2006
30. Yen MT, Pflugfelder SC, Feuer WJ (2001) The effect of punctal occlusion on tear production, tear clearance, and ocular surface sensation in normal subjects. Am J Ophthalmol 131:314–323
31. Paulsen F, Berry M (2006) Mucins and TFF peptides of the tear film and lacrimal apparatus. Prog Histochem Cytochem 41:1–53
32. Paulsen FP, Schandig U, Fabian A, Ehrich D, Sels (2006) TFF peptides and mucins are major components of dacryoliths. Graefes Arch Clin Exp Ophthalmol 244:1160–1170

Chapter 3

Diagnostics

P. Komínek, R.C. Della Rocca and S. Rosenbaum

3

Core Messages

- The proper clinical evaluation of a lacrimal function and lacrimal anatomy is an essential pre-condition for suitable therapy.
- The surgeon should be able to answer whether surgery is indicated, and if that is so, the surgery should be directed at the lacrimal apparatus, the eyelids, and punctum, or both.
- Evaluation of the lacrimal system, i.e. history, palpation, FDT, syringing and proviny, may readily yield definitive results; however, at times, more testing, including radiography, may be neccesary to arrive at a specific diagnosis and subsequent recommendations.
- Nuclear lacrimal scintigraphy is useful only in those patients whose lacrimal system is patent to syringing.
- Dacryocystography and scintigraphy are not mutually exclusive but instead complement each other.

Contents

3.1 Introduction

Two basic causes of tearing exist, epiphora associated with blockage of the lacrimal system, and excess lacrimation which is less frequent. Lacrimation (hypersecretion, reflex tearing, hyperlacrimation) is excessive tearing caused by reflex hypersecretion due to the irritation of the cornea or conjunctiva [9, 12, 19]. Unilateral lacrimation is caused by trigeminal sensory nerve stimulation in corneal diseases, i.e., corneal foreign body, abrasion, keratitis, etc. Bilateral lacrimation is typically chronic and is typically associated with chronic or recurrent conjunctivitis, staphylococcal lid margin diseases (blepharitis), and ocular surface diseases (dry eye).

Epiphora is tearing caused by a reduced tear transport or defective tear drainage outflow, i.e., epiphora is a result of a failure of tear drainage [8, 12, 14, 20]. Epiphora is caused by mechanical obstruction to the lacrimal drainage system which may include puncta, canaliculi, lacrimal sac, or nasolacrimal duct obstruction. The second, but less frequent, cause is lacrimal pump failure due to lower lid laxity or weakness of the orbicularis muscle [12, 22]. Epiphora due to obstruction can occur bilaterally especially in patients with significant sinusitis [12].

Epiphora can be caused by congenital and acquired diseases, i.e., congenital nasolacrimal duct obstructions in children, primary acquired nasolacrimal duct obstructions (PANDO), dacryocystolithiasis, orbital and lacrimal trauma, canalicular lacerations, actinomyces within the canaliculi, and canalicular obstruction following herpetic infections, ectropion, etc.

Symptoms of epiphora may range from a sensation of intermittent wetness in the eye to the permanent tear overflowing onto the cheek. Unilateral tearing is felt more intensively than bilateral tearing. Epiphora is typically worse in winter and windy weather (Table 3.1), and the incidence of epiphora increases with age [22].

The main and essential goal of examination is to distinguish between epiphora and lacrimation. While epiphora is treated mostly with surgical procedures, the lacrimation is treated mostly with medical therapy [12, 14].

Table 3.1. Epiphora grading

Grade I	Temporary epiphora outside in cold and windy weather
Grade II	Permanent epiphora outside
Grade III	Permanent epiphora outside and inside

3.1.1 Terminology

Differentiation between anatomical obstructions and functional disorders (dysfunctions) of the lacrimal system is required before beginning a treatment plan:

- Anatomical obstructions are those in which some pathological changes and irregularity in the lacrimal drainage system are found, i.e., canalicular stenosis, canalicular blockade, lacrimal sac deformation, obstruction of the nasolacrimal duct, diverticulus, etc. The lacrimal system can be changed primarily in inflammation of the lining inside the lacrimal pathways, *intrinsic*, or the lacrimal pathways can be secondarily changed from the outside, *extrinsic*, i.e., lymphoid tumor lying around the lacrimal sac. Anatomical disorders are more common than functional ones.
- Physiological dysfunction, functional epiphora is caused by disorders in which tearing does not result from anatomical changes of the lacrimal pathways themselves, but from a failure of functional lacrimal pump mechanism. It can be caused by the anatomic abnormality outside the lacrimal pathways, such as eyelid malpositions within the eyelids, punctal eversion, or lacrimal pump insufficiency caused by poor orbicularis muscle tone or eyelid laxity as seen in the paretic eyelid caused by Bell's palsy.

The locations are as follows:

1. Suprasaccal (presaccular): occurs proximal to the lacrimal sac, e.g., obstruction in the upper or lower canaliculi or common canaliculus, for example, following herpetic infection, trauma, post-irradiation, etc. (Fig. 3.1).Saccal (saccular) – occur in the lacrimal sac, e.g., diverticulus, trauma, tumor, etc.
2. Subsaccal (nasolacrimal duct, postsaccular): occurs in the nasolacrimal duct; those obstructions are most common, e.g., a congenital nasolacrimal duct obstruction, primary acquired nasolacrimal duct obstruction (PANDO), nasolacrimal duct obstruction following func-

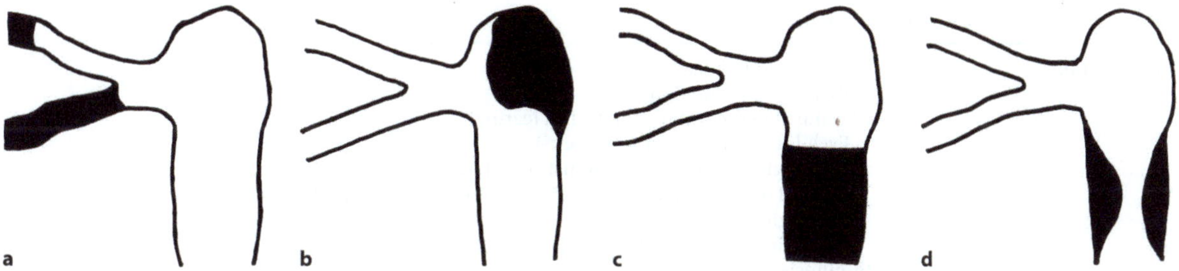

Fig. 3.1. Essential kinds of lacrimal system obstructions. a Suprasaccal obstruction. b Saccal obstruction. c Subsaccal complete obstruction. d Nasolacrimal duct stenosis. (From [14])

tional endoscopic sinus surgery, etc. Dacryocystorhinostomy is indicated in the majority of these cases.

A controversial term, *functional obstruction*, is sometimes used for findings in which the system is patent to syringing in a patient complaining of tearing; however, some anatomical pathologies in the lacrimal system are usually found in dacryocystography and other anatomical tests are needed. It is important to bear in mind that if a system is patent to syringing, it does not mean that it is normal and the drainage function may not be working under normal physiological conditions, e.g., lacrimal system is in stenosis of nasolacrimal duct patent for syringing with a higher hydrostatic pressure, but under usual conditions there is an insufficient drainage (it can be determined with fluorescein test or with nuclear scintigraphy). That is why the term "obstruction" should be used only for anatomical disorders and the term "functional obstruction" should not be used in this sense [12].

3.2 Diagnostics Philosophy

Tearing can be caused by hypersecretion and epiphora, both of which can be combined. Clinical symptoms occur if the balance between the tear production and drainage function of lacrimal system has changed, i.e., the clinical picture of epiphora does not depend on the absolute functional status of either one [9, 14]. That is why there are no symptoms of epiphora if lacrimal production is reduced and lacrimal drainage is decreased, e.g., in older patients, etc. (Table 3.2).

The basic diagnostic evaluation of the tearing patient should include quantification of tear production and assessment of nasolacrimal system patency [21]. The goals of history and clinical examinations of patients are to define pathological processes responsible for tearing present, to distinguish anatomical and functional epiphora and, in an anatomical obstruction, to identify the level at which the obstruction lies and its extension as well [24]. One should be able to determine *whether surgery is indicated and whether the surgery will be directed in the lacrimal apparatus, the eyelids, or punctum, or both* [9].

The goals of the examination of tearing patients are as follows:

- Distinguish epiphora and lacrimation
- Define pathological process responsible for tearing
- Distinguish anatomical and functional disorders
- Evaluate block location and its extent, and define a surgical approach

There are a lot of clinical diagnostic tests, many of which must be used together in order to diagnose specific disease processes adequately. The choice of tests should be logical enough to reveal the cause of an obstruction and to recommend a proper therapy [9]. The tests are divided into the following categories:

- Anatomical: tests for investigation of morphological disordes and location of obstruction (Table 3.3)
- Functional (physiological): tests for drainage lacrimal function under normal condition (if there is no obstruction and no higher pressure as in syringing).
- Secretion: tests for assessment of secretion (used in the examination of dry eye)

Table 3.2. Typical causes of epiphora and lacrimation

Lacrimation	Supranuclear (CNS) Psychogenic (emotions, etc.) Trigeminal nerve stimulation (reflex tearing) Eyelids (blepharitis, trichiasis, etc.) Conjunctival diseases (inflammation, a foreign body, etc.) Corneal diseases (dry eye, a foreign body, contact lens, etc.) Neuralgic (neuralgia) Ocular inflammation (iritis, etc.) Infranuclear Facial nerve abberant innervation, crocodile tears Lacrimal gland stimulation Others Bright lights, sneezing, etc.
Epiphora	Functional (lacrimal pump insufficiency) Incorrect eyelid closure (orbicularis muscle laxity, lagophthalmus, trauma, following surgery, etc.) Eyelid malposition: ectropion and entropion (involutional, mechanical, cicatricial) Punctal eversion, punctal medialization Anatomical lacrimal system obstructions (stenosis and obliterations) Punctal and canalicular (congenital, inflammation; herpetic, traumatic, idiopathic, chronic lid ectropion, burns, pharmacological, etc.) Saccal (inflammation, sarcoidosis, tumors, trauma, etc.) Nasolacrimal duct (congenital obstruction, primary acquired obstruction-PANDO, trauma, tumor, etc.) Nasal (hay fever, rhinosinusitis, surgery, tumors, etc.)
Combined lacrimation (L) + epiphora (E)	Combinations 1+2 Facial nerve palsy Lagophthalmus (L), corneal irritation (E), lacrimal pump dysfunction (E) Involutional lower lid entropion Corneal irritation from the inturning lid and lashes (L), ineffective lacrimal pump (E) Lower lid ectropion Conjunctival irritation (L), ineffective lacrimal pump (E) Thyroid diseases Corneal irritation (L), defective canalicular function (E)

Table 3.3. Clinical tests in a tearing patient

Epiphora		Lacrimation
Anatomical tests	Physiological tests	Test of secretion
Palpation of the lacrimal sac	Fluorescein dye disappearance	Schirmer's test
Syringing (irrigation)	Scintigraphy	Bengal rose test
Diagnostic probing	Jones dye I	Tear-film break-up
Dacryocystography	Sacharin test	Tear lysozyme
Nasal examination		
CT, MRI		

The diagnosis is usually made by ophthalmologists. The otorhinolaryngologists who participate in a nasal examination and lacrimal surgical therapy should, however, know the principles of tests and should be able to identify the level and extension of the obstruction.

3.3 Examination

The diagnostic tests used for evaluating the nasolacrimal system are done after an ophthalmological examination which has excluded the ocular surface diseases and inflammatory diseases as causes of epiphora [25]. The examination may be sometimes very easy and epiphora diagnostic can be made on history only. The determination of its etiology, however, may be exteremely difficult and often requires a variety of diagnostic procedures [9, 14, 28].

Studies of the lacrimal system should be done bilaterally whenever possible, as this may help to differentiate [25]. The tests vary in the extent to which they evaluate the anatomy and physiology of the lacrimal drainage system.

3.3.1 Clinical History

An accurate history is one of the most important aspects in the evaluation of the patients with tearing. The history and external examinations may provide important clues as to the presence of canalicular disease [26]. The history must incorporate the patient's present and past ophthalmic symptoms, nasal symptoms, as well as medical and interventional histories with special attention given to glaucoma medications. The intermittency and the duration of tearing is important. One must ascertain the significance of the tearing prior to making a decision to recommend surgical repair.

Unilateral tearing often indicates a local obstructive, traumatic, inflammatory, or infectious process in the drainage pathways, whereas bilateral tearing may denote excess secretion due to an allergic response, iritis, or keratoconjunctivitis. Constant tearing is more likely associated with the causes of unilateral tearing, whereas intermittent tearing is more common in patients with problems causing secondary unilateral or bilateral tearing.

Epiphora in a child with a history of tearing since birth has been caused mostly by an obstructive membrane within the naso-lacrimal duct (Valve of Hasner). Intermittent acquired epiphora in an adult usually results from partial stenosis of the membranous duct and/or dacryolithiasis, and may also be seen in patients with allergic rhinitis. The relationship of symptoms to the previous medical therapy (topical idoxuridine, phospholine iodide, systemic 5-fluorouracil), orbital trauma, and environmental factors, however, as to the head position, stress, etc., are also factors. Previous sinus surgery should indicate the possibility of duct injury as well. The presence of recurrent sinus disease can cause rhinitis or intranasal polyps.

3.3.2 External Examination and Palpation

A careful history must be combined with the external exmination of the lacrimal system that begins with an inspection of the face, external ocular surface, and eyelid structure including the position and contour of the eyelid and eye blink (Table 3.4). Periorbital and facial asymmetry are looked for, as well as the lid malposition, bulges in the medial canthal area, facial nerve palsy, etc.

Table 3.4. Watering patients: external inspection and palpation

Eyelids	Lower lid laxity, ectropion, entropion, punctal eversion, trichiasis, blepharitis, snap-back test, pinch test, etc.
Medial canthus	Lacrimal sac enlargement below the medial canthal tendon (acute dacryoccystitis, mucocele, etc.), enlargement above the medial canthal tendon (neoplasm)
Palpation of the lacrimal sac	Reflux of mucopurulent material (mucocoele with an obstruction at the lower end of the sac or in the lacrimal duct and a patent canalicular system, or an obstruction of lower or upper canaliculi), pressure over the sac in acute dacryocystitis causes pain

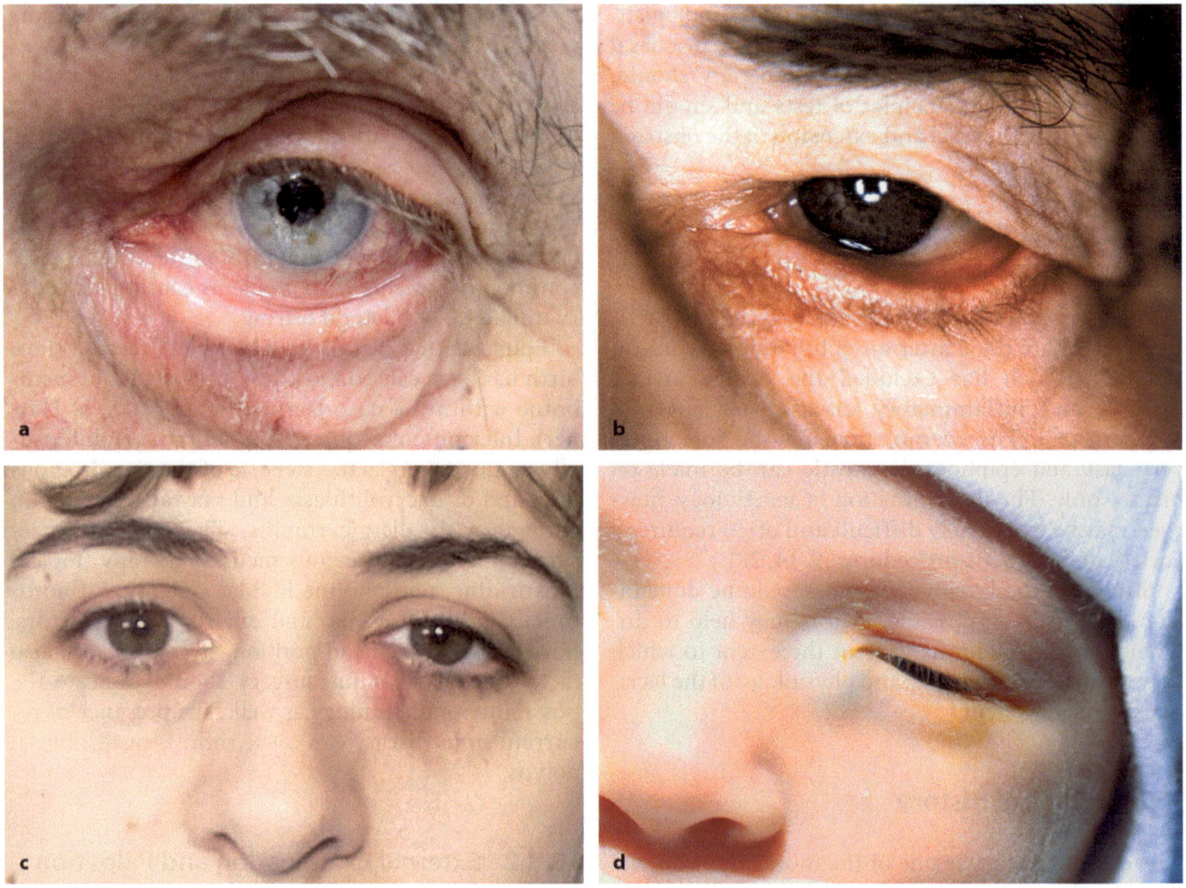

Fig. 3.2. External examination. a Involutional ectropion, a right medial ectropion with a dry inferior punctum. b Patient with facial palsy and severe lid laxity paralytic ectropion. c Red mass below the medial canthal tendon (acute dacryocystitis, treated with endonasal dacryocystorhinostomy). d Amniotocele in a newborn (From [14])

A slit-lamp examination is essential to determine a position of the upper punctum in relation to the lower punctum on blinking and a change in the position between the upper and lower eyelid, and to see if there is any lagophthalmus or evidence of orbicularis dysfunction [1, 9, 20]. The puncta should face slightly towards the lacrimal lake. The puncta, normally 0.3 mm in diameter, may appear phimotic, causing obstruction [7]. If puncta are present and open, the discharge from the puncta is sought. The papilla and eyelids along the canaliculi, if red or swollen, may indicate canaliculitis. Canaliculitis may be confirmed by expressing yellow cheesy material from the canaliculi by pressing on the swelling canaliculus with a cotton bud. This is not possible if there is severe tenderness. The absence of puncta may be a congenital trait or evidence of previous inflammatory diseases.

A slit-lamp examination can reveal inferior punctate corneal staining, and epithelial filaments suggests an inadequate tear meniscus. There should be a 1-mm marginal tear strip along the lower lid, between the globe and lid margin. The size and character of the tear meniscus can be important. A small strip of fluorescein can be applied to the inferior fornix. The absence of any tear strip is suggestive of a dry eye syndrome. Conjunctival or corneal irritation, either inflammatory or mechanical, may cause hypersecretion with the resultant epiphora. Marginal blepharitis is a common condition associated with the increased lacrimation. In the absence of inflammation, an increased tear meniscus is indicative of naso lacrimal duct obstruction.

Lid laxity with ectropion may lead to the corneal exposure and reflex lacrimal oversecretion, or to a physiological dysfunction due to a weakened orbicularis pump mechanism or punctal eversion (Figs. 3.2, 3.4).

The resiliency of the lid can be measured with the snap-back test [9, 20]. The lower lid is pulled down away from the globe, then released, and the speed with which the lid "snaps back" against the globe is observed, as well as whether there is a short gap between the lid and globe (Fig. 3.4).

Horizontal eyelid laxity may be estimated with the pinch test [9]. The lid is firmly pulled away from the globe and the distance between the lid and the eye is measured. More than 8 mm of distraction between the lid and the cornea is suggestive of laxity and a functional epiphora may exist.

Medial canthal tendon laxity and secondary partial or medical ectropion are assessed with the help of the lateral distraction test [20]. The lower puncta should remain in its position while the lid is pulled laterally. Up to 1–2 mm, the movement is normal in the young and adult, and up to 3–4 mm in the elderly.

Mass lesion in the medial canthal region may mechanically obstruct a lacrimal system. Redness, swelling, pain, and tenderness in the lacrimal sac area suggest an acute dacryocystitis (Fig. 3.2). Chronic dacryocysitis itself may manifest as the distention of the lacrimal sac. A normal lacrimal sac is not palpable. The lacrimal sac swelling is typically confined to the region below the medial canthal tendon; neoplasms usually extend above the tendon [14].

Mucopurulent material can be expressed through the punctum and canaliculi if the canaliculi and valve of Rosenmüller are patent and healthy, and if the lacrimal sac is palpated. It must be noted whether there is regurgitation through only one canaliculus or both; and the nature of the reflux as well: whether the reflux is clear, purulent, or bloody. The small finger is applied to the anterior lacrimal crest and rolled gently medially to expose muco-purulent reflux. When the sac or dacryocystocele is large and hard, pressure is not applied in order to minimize pain (Fig. 3.3).

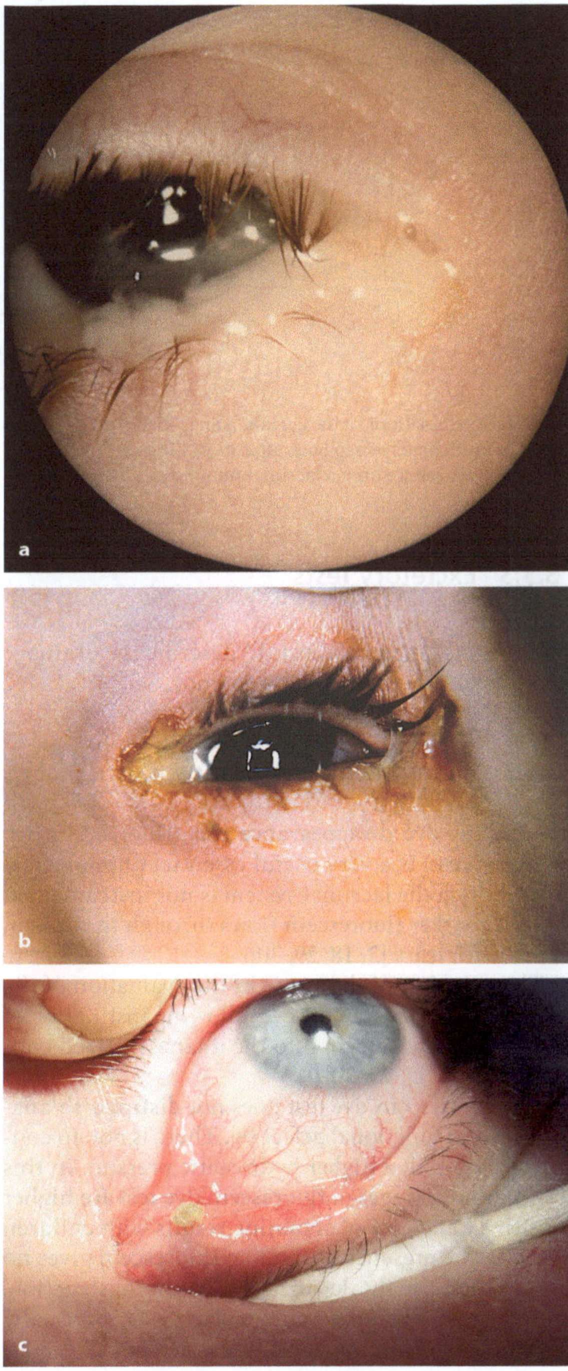

Fig. 3.3. a Mucopurulent discharge from the lacrimal system in chronic dacryocystitis. b Eczematized skin of the long-standing mucoporulent discharge of the eyelids. c Chronic lower actinomycetes canaliculisis. Canaliculitis is confirmed by expressing cheesy material from the canaliculus with a cotton bud. (From [14])

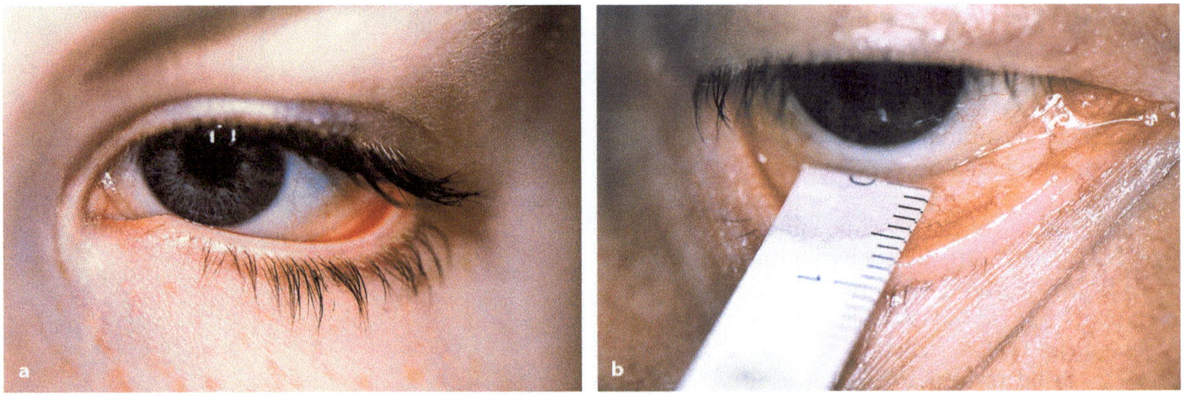

Fig. 3.4. Examinations of the eyelids. **a** Snap-back test. If the lid does not immediately snap back after its pulling downward and releasing, one can assume a lacrimal pump dysfunction. **b** Distraction test. The lid is grasped and pulled away from the globe. More than 8 mm distraction between the lid and the cornea is suggestive of laxity. (From [14])

3.3.3 Excretory Tests

The goal of excretory tests is to describe the drainage function and lacrimal system patency.

3.3.3.1 Fluorescein Dye Disappearance Test

Fluorescein dye disappearance test (fluorescein dye retention test) is a very useful essential physiological test in which the lacrimal system is not instrumented and the marker fluorescein flows through the system mixed with tears [2, 18, 29, 30].

The principle of the test is in the evaluation of the residual fluorescein in the eye following instillation of one drop of fluorescein into the unanesthetized conjunctival sac [17, 29, 30].

The fluorescein dye test does not distinguish anatomical and functional defect [9]. There is not, in contrast to Jones II, a higher hydrostatic pressure in this test. The advantages of fluorescein dye test are higher sensitivity and ease of obtaining results with children [14, 17]. The presence of residual fluorescein gives no information on the localization of the obstruction, and that is why other anatomical tests, especially probing and syringing, must be carried out (Fig. 3.5).

Performance
One drop of 0.125–2% fluorescein is instilled into the unanesthetized lower fornix of each conjunctival sac. After 5 min, the thickness of the fluorescence of the tear meniscus is measured with the help of cobalt-blue filter. The tears normally drain down the system in 5 min. The test is positive if residual fluorescein is present. In infants, the child must be placed on a parent's knee or held in arms, and the head must be in a vertical position.

The fluorescein dye test grading scale is as follows [17]:

- 0=no fluorescence in the conjunctival sac
- 1=thin fluorescing marginal tear strip persists
- 2=more fluorescein persists, between 1 and 3
- 3=wide, brighly fluorescing tear strip

Grades 0 and 1 are considered to be normal, i.e., the drainage function is good. Grades 2 and 3 are considered to be abnormal and the lacrimal drainage system is not functional.

False-negative findings may occur due to a large lacrimal sac or mucocele, or a distal nasolacrimal duct block, where the dye with fluorescein can pool in the sac or duct [19].

If a drop of fluorescein is placed in the external canthus on the lower eyelid, its transport can be observed from lateral to medial across the eyelid and into each punctum, and the holes in the tear film can be observed (break-up time test).

Fluorescein may be sought in the nose if a patient is asked to blow the nose or the nose is examined endoscopically.

In most patients with epiphora the history, palpation, and inspection, fluorescein dye disappearance

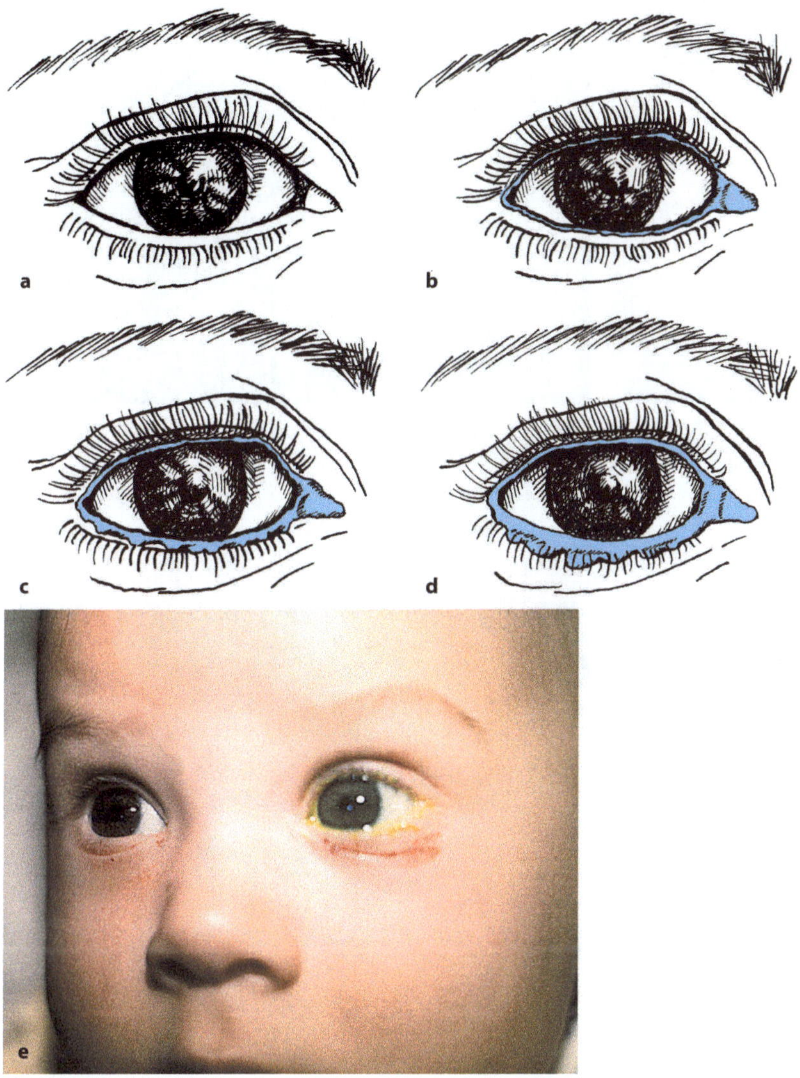

Fig. 3.5. Fluorescein dye disappearance test. **a** Grade 0=no fluorescence in the conjunctival sac. **b** Grade 1=thin fluorescing marginal tear strips only. **c** Grade 2=between 1 and 2. **d** Grade 3=brightly fluorescing tear strip. **e** Asymmetry in test: retention of fluorescein on the left side in a congenital nasolacrimal obstruction. (From [14])

test, diagnostic probing, and irrigation of the nasolacrimal system is sufficient for the determination of the drainage function, location, and degree of anatomical block.

3.3.3.2 Jones Fluorescein Tests and Saccharine Test

Jones tests are rarely used because of their false negativity and the fluorescein dye test is preferred [9, 20, 29, 30]. Jones tests can be performed only if the lacrimal system is patent for syringing, i.e., there is no complete obstruction in the lacrimal system. The primary dye test is a physiological test, and although it is limited, it has some benefit [9].

Saccharin test is a physiological test similar to fluorescein dye test [7]. A drop of saccharin is placed into the anesthetized conjunctival sac and the time is measured until the patient tastes saccharin (approximately 3.5 min; patients should not have any problem with tasting). As the test cannot be used in small children (in comparison with fluorescein dye test) and gives us no anatomical information, we do not use it.

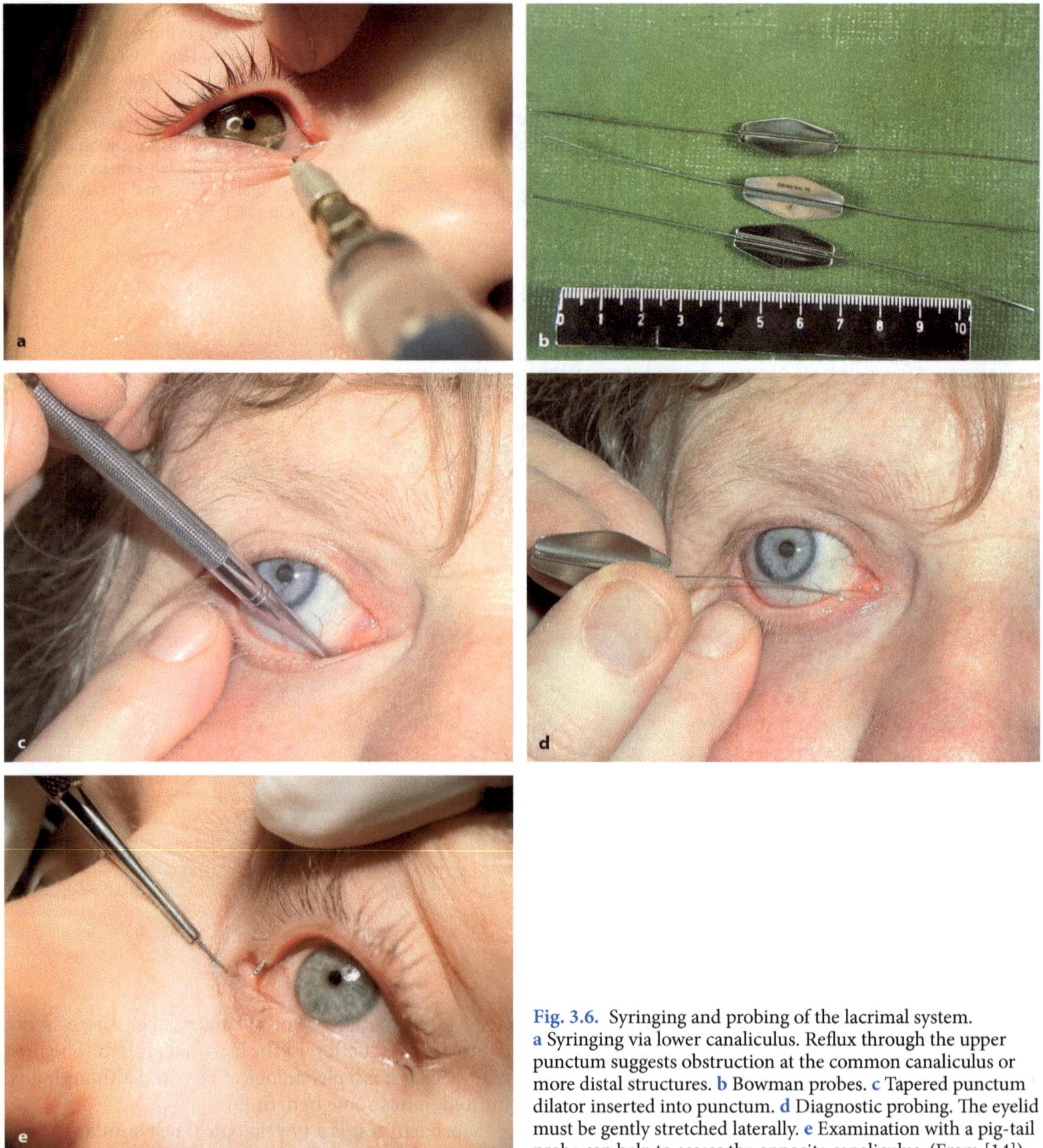

Fig. 3.6. Syringing and probing of the lacrimal system. a Syringing via lower canaliculus. Reflux through the upper punctum suggests obstruction at the common canaliculus or more distal structures. b Bowman probes. c Tapered punctum dilator inserted into punctum. d Diagnostic probing. The eyelid must be gently stretched laterally. e Examination with a pig-tail probe can help to assess the opposite canaliculus. (From [14])

3.4 Diagnostic Probing and Lacrimal Syringing (Irrigating)

The irrigation and diagnostic probing of the proximal lacrimal drainage system are essential anatomical tests giving very valuable information on the presence, location, and form obstruction. They may qualitatively establish patency or stenosis of the canaliculi, lacrimal sac, and nasolacrimal duct, but they are not able to provide any information on functional insufficiency [22].

3.4.1 Syringing: Irrigation

The syringing is not a physiological test because of using a higher hydrostatic pressure than the normal tear outflow [12]. The information resulting from the tests is to be interpreted in connection with the fluorescein dye test and clinical examination (Fig. 3.6).

3.4.1.1 Performance

The following steps are taken:

1. After several applications of topical anesthetic have been instilled, the punctum and ampulla are dilated with a punctal dilator in case the puncta are small. The punctum and proximal canaliculae can be stabilized with a finger on the lower eyelid retracting the lid inferiorly.
2. A blunt cannula is placed in the inferior canaliculus and the lower eyelid is pulled down and laterally in order to straighten the lower canaliculus and evert the punctum away from the ocular surface. The superior canaliculus is gently stretched laterally prior to irrigation.
3. The tip of the irrigator is placed in the inferior canaliculus, first vertically and then horizontally with the eyelid on stretch. The tip is advanced 3–7 mm into the canaliculus and sterile water or saline is used as an irrigant.

It is important to avoid forced irrigation to limit injury to canaliculi and to obtain more accurate analysis of patency, delayed patency or obstruction. If the inferior punctum is absent or there is a canalicular obstruction, the syringing is repeated via the upper punctum. For the upper punctum irrigation the patient is asked to look down and laterally while the canaliculus is stretched laterally and is slightly everted.

3.4.1.2 Syringing: Interpretation

Reflux (regurgitation) through the opposite punctum suggests an obstruction in the common canaliculus or more distal structures. Fluid coming directly back through the same punctum indicates a canalicular obstruction and the syringing must be repeated through the opposite canaliculus. Distention of the lacrimal sac implies an obstruction of the nasolacrimal duct. Irrigation into the nose indicates an anatomically patent system but not necessarily a functional system.

Partial irrigation into the nose accompanied by some amount of reflux indicates a partial obstruction. It is necessary to assesss whether the water passes into thc nose, back out the upper canaliculus, back out the lower canaliculus, or some combination thereof. If there is an obstruction of one or both canaliculi, the length of residual canaliculus proximal to the obstruction should be measured.

Patency to syringing by itself does not mean that the lacrimal drainage system is normal and does not involve lacrimal functioning, and thus other tests must be run to determine the cause of epiphora before surgery [14, 21]. Avoid probing or irrigation if signs of accute dacryocystitis exist.

3.5 Diagnostic Probing

Probing is generally performed only if the syringing and other tests demonstrate an obstruction and the location and extension of the obstruction is to be described (Table 3.5). The obstructions may be located in the canaliculi and their assessment is an essential goal in patients with epiphora. If fluid regurgitates through the opposite punctum, the obstruction of common canaliculus or more distal structures are suggested and it must be distinguished between them with probing.

Probing can be made with blunt long curved lacrimal cannula for syringe or with Bowman probe. We prefer Bowman probes because of their different sizes, better holding in the hand, and better sensitivity in handling canaliculi. If signs of dacryocystitis with the

Table 3.5. Syringing and probing via the lower canaliculus

	Pharynx and nose	Reflux lower canaliculus	Reflux upper canaliculus	Lacrimal system results
Hard stop	Yes	No	No	Normal
	Yes	No	Yes	Nasolacrimal duct stenosis
	No	No	Yes	Subsaccal obstruction (usually mucoid or mucopurulent discharge)
Soft stop	No	Yes	No	Medial canalicular or common canaliculus block
	No	No	Yes	Distal common canaliculus block

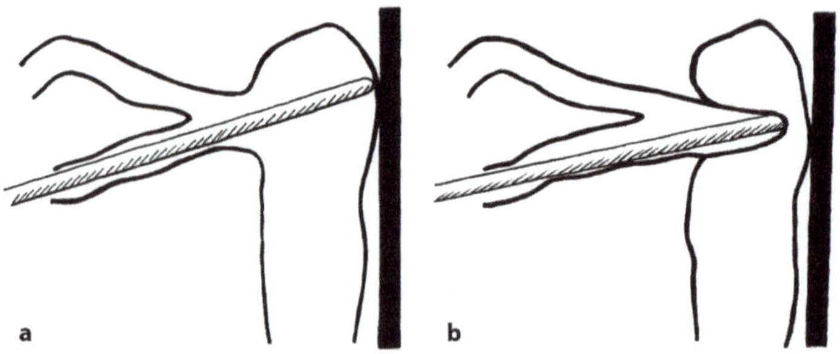

Fig. 3.7. Hard and soft stops. **a** Hard stop: the probe passed into the sac touches its medial wall, and the common canaliculus is patent. **b** Soft stop: spongy feeling; the probe presses the common canaliculus against the medial wall of the sac. A medial shift in the inner canthus is observed from the outside. (From [14])

presence of mucopurulent reflux exist when digital pressure is applied to the anterior the anterior crest and lateral to the crest, neither irrigation nor probing are required.

3.5.1 Performance

After topical anesthetic is instilled, the punctum is dilated and an appropriately sized lacrimal probe is advanced into the canaliculus. First the probe is passed vertically through the punctum and then horizontally with the eyelid on a stretch until it encounters the lacrimal bone or meets the canalicular obstruction.

If the probe (lacrimal cannula) is advanced into the canaliculus and encounters the lacrimal bone, the feeling is called "hard stop", i.e., it is suggested that the probe passed into the sac, touched its medial wall, and the common canaliculus is patent (Fig. 3.7). If there was a reflux through the opposite punctum in syringing a "hard stop" suggests an obstruction of the sac or duct.

If there is canalicular block, the length of the advanced probe is measured and this length accords with the patent proximal part of canaliculi, i.e. the distance between the punctum and obstruction is measured. It is necessary to evaluate the opposite canaliculus as well.

If there is an obstruction near to the lacrimal sac and the probe cannot pass into the lacrimal sac to a "hard stop," one feels a "soft stop." This spongy feeling suggests that the obstruction is probably within the common canaliculus and the lacrimal probe (cannula) presses the common canaliculus and the lateral wall against the medial wall of the sac. The probing must be done in a very gentle way. It is useful to look at the inner canthus while one is advancing the probe toward the hard stop. If the obstruction is not in canaliculi and the probe is in the lacrimal sac, the inner canthus should not shift. If there is a medial shift in the inner canthus in advancing the probe toward the lacrimal bone, it indicates that the probe is dragging the common canaliculus medially toward the bone and the lacrimal bone has not yet been reached. The differentiation between the hard stop and soft stop is essential because the treatment an obstruction at the sac or duct versus the common canaliculus requires different DCR techniques (Table 3.5).

Hard stop is a firm feeling of the medial bone bordering the lacrimal sac in canalicular probing. It usually excludes a complete obstruction to the canalicular system. Soft stop is a spongy feeling that indicates a common canaliculus obstruction as the probe presses the common canaliculus and the lateral wall against the medial wall of the sac. A medial shift observed in the inner canthus signifies that the lacrimal bone has not yet been reached with the probe.

It is important to have a mental image of what the findings taken from probing and syringing look like, and it is useful to record this on an outline of the lacrimal system.

3.6 Radiological Examination

Radiological tests are to be performed if the decision as to the method of treatment cannot be made without any radiological information [8, 11]. Radiological examinations include dacryocystography (DCG), nuclear lacrimal scintigraphy, computed tomography (CT), and magnetic resonance imaging (MRI).

Dacryocystography is an anatomical investigation and is indicated if there is a block on syringing in the lacrimal system, and thus it can help in creating an image of how the internal anatomy of the lacrimal system looks. Scintigraphy is a functional test and is useful in assessing the site of a delayed tear transit, i. e., it is useful only if the lacrimal system is patent on syringing. Both CT and MRI are used very seldom and are reserved only for some patients with preceded trauma, facial surgery, tumor, or in whom sinus diseases are suspected.

It is important to correlate the results of radiological investigations with those of the other tests and investigations. The difficulty of radiological tests of the lacrimal system is the tendency to consider the information obtained from an anatomical test to be of a functional nature, and to consider the information received from a functional test to indicate a specific anatomical defect.

3.6.1 Dacryocystography

Dacryocystography is a method in which injection of the radio-opaque water-soluble fluid is instilled into either lower or upper canaliculus taking magnified images. The digital subtraction technique is preferred because it gives an image of better quality (Fig. 3.8).

A DCG better evaluates the lacrimal sac and duct anatomy, but it evaluates worse canalicular anatomy. It outlines diverticulae and fistulae, and shows intrasac pathology (dacryoliths or tumor) and the sac size.

A DCG is not routinely performed [9–11, 14, 16]. It is seldom necessary with a complete obstruction in the non-traumatic situation. It can be especially useful in patients with previous trauma to localize the position of bone fragments or, after previously unsuccessful lacrimal surgery, to determine the size of the sac. With patency to syringing, the DCG helps to determine whether the stenosis is in the common canaliculus or sac, and it can rule out the presence of a lacrimal sac diverticulum [10]. A DCG can often find drainage abnormalities present in patients with "functional obstruction" [10].

3.6.2 Indications for Dacryocystography

The indications for dacryocystography are as follows:

1. Complete obstructions: the size of the sac; determination of the exact location of an obstruction (common canaliculus, sac)
2. Incomplete obstructions and intermitent tearing: location of the stenosis; diverticuli; stones; and no anatomical pathology (functional disorders)
3. Failed lacrimal surgery: size of the sac
4. Suspicion of sac tumors

3.6.2.1 Performance

The DCG is performed in the supine position under topical anesthesia. The puncta are dilated and a canula (irrigation canula) attached with syringe containing a water-soluble contrast medium is inserted and taped into position. After an intracanalicular injection under pressure, a film is taken.

Bilateral studies give a chance to compare both sides [10].

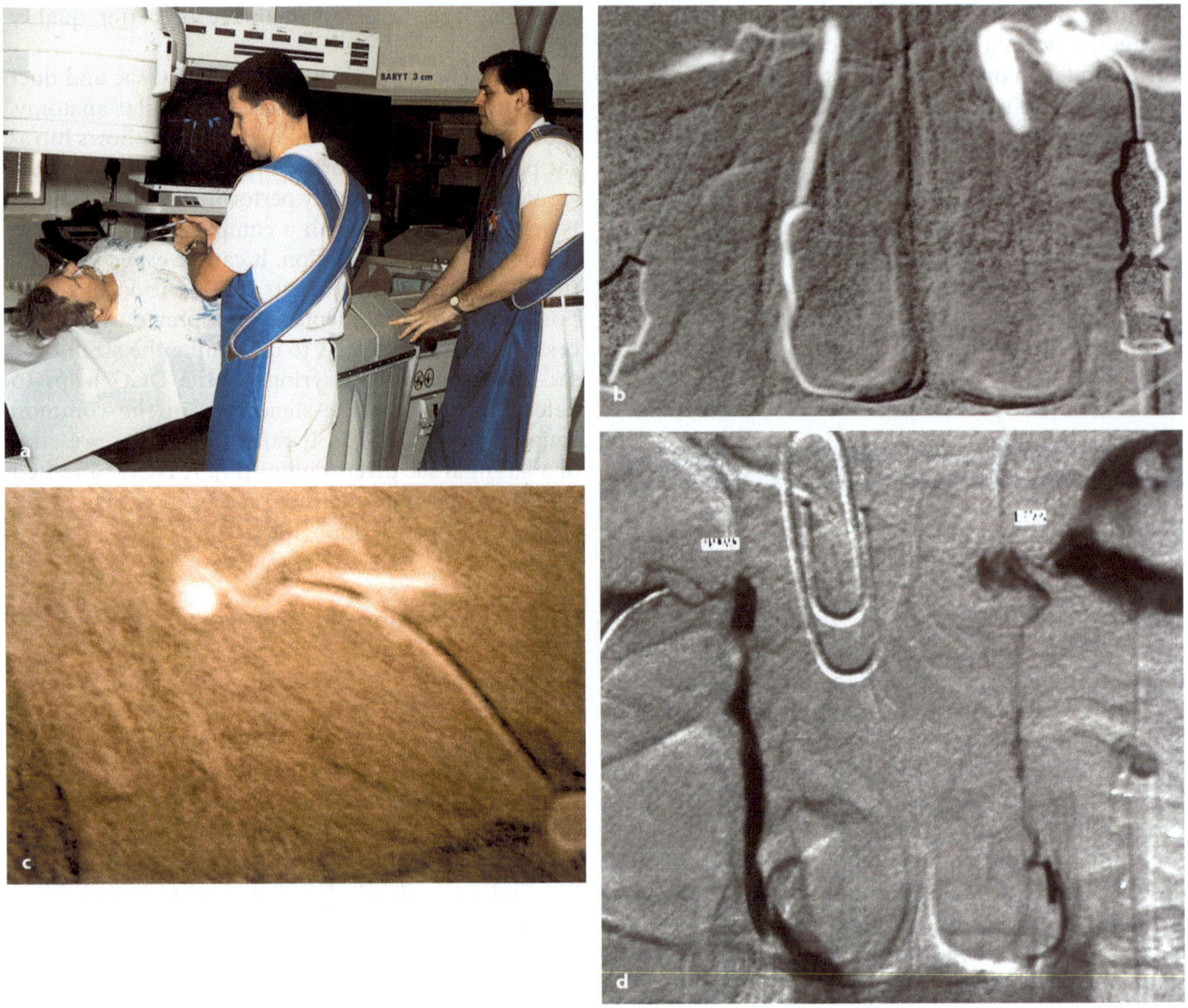

Fig. 3.8. Digital subtraction dacryocystography (DCG). **a** A DCG set-up. Patient lying on a bed; contrast material injection is given by examiners. **b** Normal lacrimal system on the right and dilated lacrimal sac with the complete obliteration at sac–duct junction on the left side. **c** Dacryocystography. Patient with a left-sided obstruction following dacryocystorhinostomy: a tiny sac is visualized. **d** A 35-year-old patient with intermitent tearing. The dacryocystogram demonstrates defect, and prestenotic dilatation of the sac on the left side indicates a stone; this was confirmed at DCR surgery

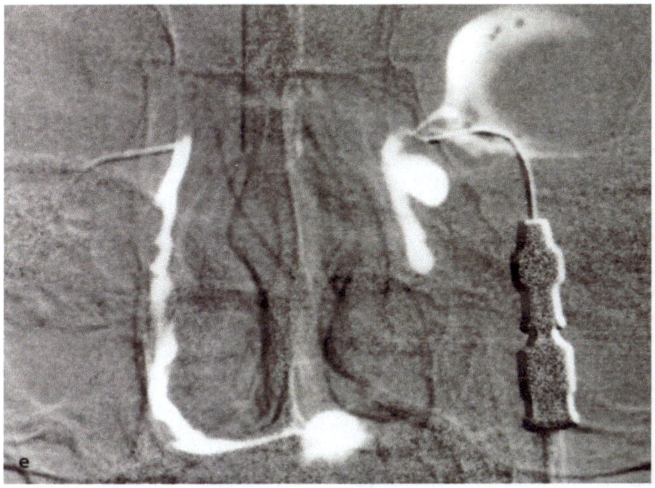

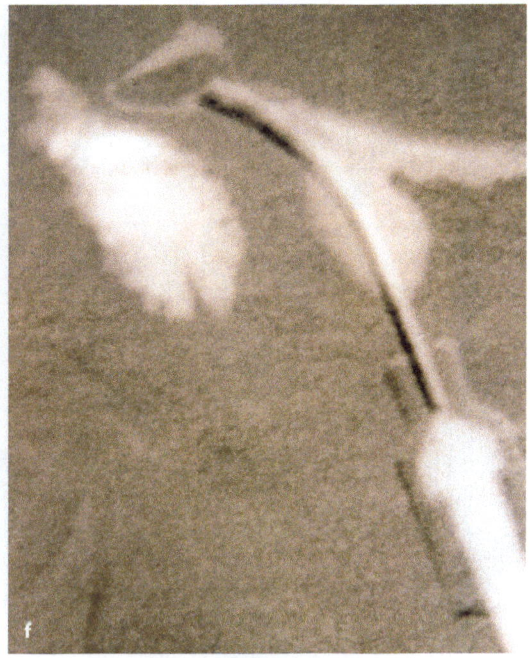

Fig. 3.8. (*Continued*) **e** Diverticulum of the lacrimal sac. **f** Dilation of the lacrimal sac on the left side in chronic dacryocystitis with an irregularity in contrast. A stone was found at DCR surgery. (From [14])

3.6.3 Radiological Criteria for Lacrimal Pathology

The radiological criteria for lacrimal pathology are as follows [22, 23]:

1. Regurgitation of (radio-opaque) fluid into the conjunctival sac (retention of fluid, absence of fluid in the nose, fluctuation of lumen of lacrimal system)
2. Irregularity in contrast
3. Cystic dilation and aneurysm
4. Deformation and drawing of the lacrimal sac

3.6.4 Nuclear Lacrimal Scintigraphy

Nuclear lacrimal scintigraphy is a simple, non-invasive physiological test that evaluates patency of the lacrimal system. Scintigraphy uses a radiotracer (technetium-99m pertechnetate), which is very easily detectable with a gamma camera (Fig. 3.9).

While a DCG is usually preferred especially in a complete obstruction, scintigraphy is useful only in those patients whose lacrimal system is patent to syringing in the presence of constant epiphora. The test is more physiological than DCG, anatomical information is lacking, and fine anatomical details are not available in comparison with DCG [9]. Correlation of the anatomical study (DCG) and functional study (scintigraphy) may be necessary in planning surgery [20]; however, it is important to bear in mind that a normal result is considered to be a contraindication to any surgical intervention [9, 14, 27].

Nuclear lacrimal scan has been found to be helpful especially in difficult cases with incompletely obstructed pathways in which DCG could not be interpreted in a safisfactory manner to determine whether surgery should be undertaken or not [11].

3.6.4.1 Performance

A drop ot technetium-99m is instilled into each conjunctival sac of a patient sitting in front of a gamma camera. No topical anesthesia is required, and normal blinking is allowed.

The patient stares at a distant target during a 20-min test for a qualitative analysis, in the course of which images are recorded (immediately following instillation, after 3, 5, 10, 15, and 20 min).

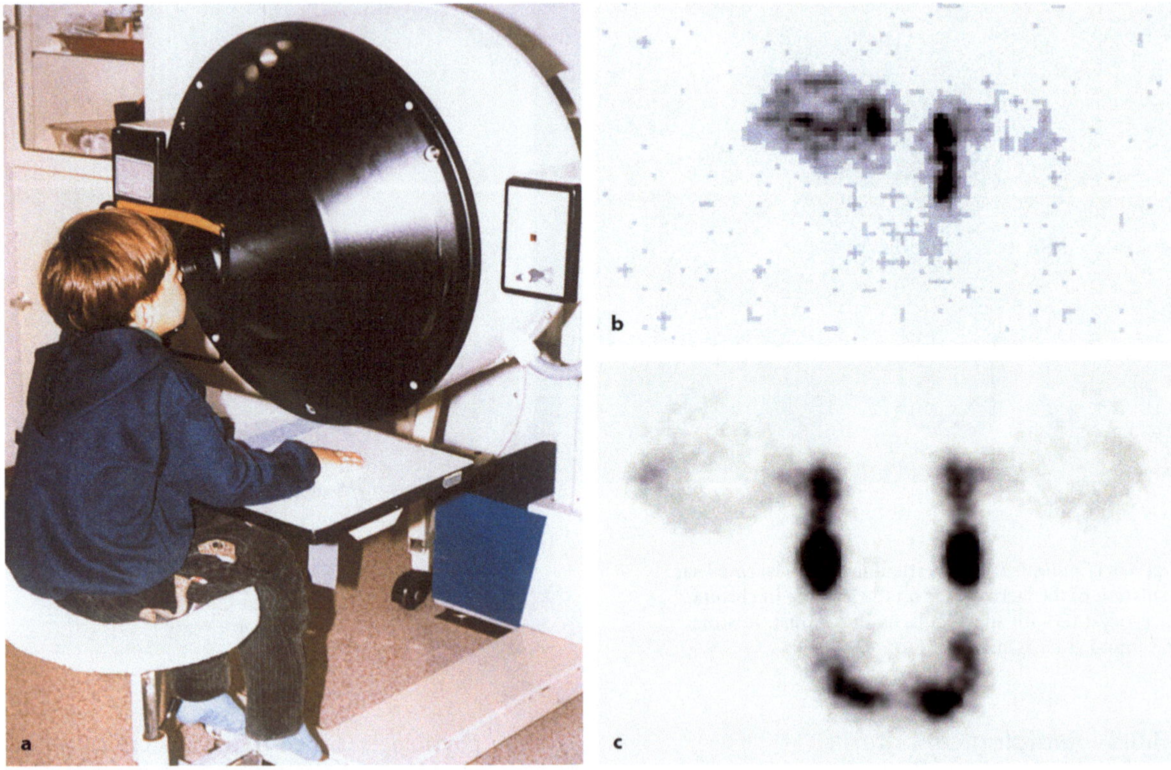

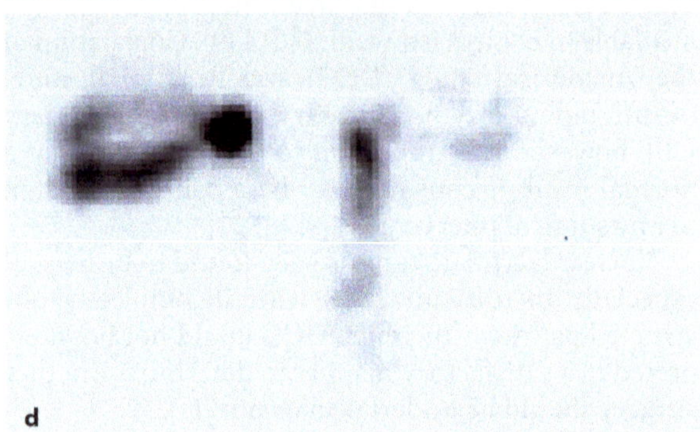

Fig. 3.9. Nuclear lacrimal scintigraphy. a Set-up for nuclear lacrimal scan. The patients sits upright with the head fixed in front of the pinhole collimator of a gamma camera. Serial images are taken as the tracer passes through the system. b Patients with right-sided tearing and patency to syringing and nasolacrimal duct stenosis on dacryocystogram. Scan after 10 min. c Normal scintigraphy. d Scan after 20 min demonstrates significant decreased flow on the right and normal flow on the left. (From [14])

A quantitative, region-of-interest analysis can be obtained as well. There are pre-saccal, sac/nasolacrimal duct junction, nasolacrimal duct, and nasal cavity areas of interest. The analysis gives percentage of drainage in mentioned areas with time and can assist in determining the area of pathology.

3.6.4.2 Nuclear Lacrimal Scan Indication

The nuclear lacrimal scan indications are as follows:

1. Interpretation of anatomical tests: if it is not possible to determine the full patency of lacrimal system or functional significant stenosis, surgery is indicated
2. Questionable lid laxity, punctal stenosis, facial nerve palsy: evaluation of lacrimal pump dysfunction or significant stenosis (indicating need for eyelid surgery)
3. Questionable epiphora: evaluation of dynamics of tear drainage; determination whether the drainage system is normal or not (if normal, no surgery is indicated)

3.6.5 Computed Tomography and MRI

Computed tomography (CT) can be helpful in assessing the structures intimately associated with the nasolacrimal drainage system (Fig. 3.10). The CT scanning is used mainly when an extrinsic disease is suspected and is of great help to the patients with paranasal sinus or facial pathology associated with the lacrimal system (tumor, rhinosinusitis, facial trauma, following facial surgery, etc.) [14].

Magnetic resonance is not used in practice in lacrimal diagnostics and is reserved only for the special cases, e.g., for differentiation of masses of the lacrimal sac [5, 20].

3.7 Nasal Examination and Nasal Endoscopy

Nasal examination, especially nasal endoscopy, should be obligatory for every lacrimal patient [6, 9, 10, 14, 20, 26]. The examination of the lacrimal area with the nasal speculum and headlight provides only a poor view of this region and is not sufficient, endoscopy provides a clear diagnostic look for nasal polyps, imporant anatomic variations, tumors, and other pathological endonasal conditions such as septal deviation (Fig. 3.10).

Diagnostic nasal endoscopy is performed with a rigid endoscope or flexible endoscope which can be used without any difficulties in small children, too. The rigid endoscopes are 4-mm diameter, 0 or 30° viewing angle, and the 2.7-mm diameter endoscope can be advantageous, especially in children and some adults with narrow nasal cavities. The inferior and the middle meatus are better viewed if some decongestants are introduced into the nose.

3.7.1 Diagnostic Nasal Endoscopy

The nasal mucosa is topically decongested and anesthetized with a spray or pledges soaked with anesthetics. The patient sits or lies, and it is advantageous especially if some endonasal manipulation with forceps is assumed, e.g., in a patient's subsequent surgery.

The examination of the nasal cavity and the lateral nasal wall is performed in a systematic fashion and usually involves three steps [14]:

1. The general survey and orientation and visual inspection of the nasal vestibule, nasopharynx, inferior turbinate, lower septum, and inferior meatus (the nasolacrimal duct opening is sometimes observed).
2. Endoscope is directed at the posterior end of the middle turbinate to evaluate the spheno-ethmoidal recess and superior nasal meatus.
3. Endoscopy of the middle meatus and lateral nasal wall, including an examination of the maxillary line and the middle meatus.

However, endoscopy is very important in postoperative care and after unsuccessful lacrimal surgery, e.g., unsuccessful dacryocystorhinostomy (Table 3.6).

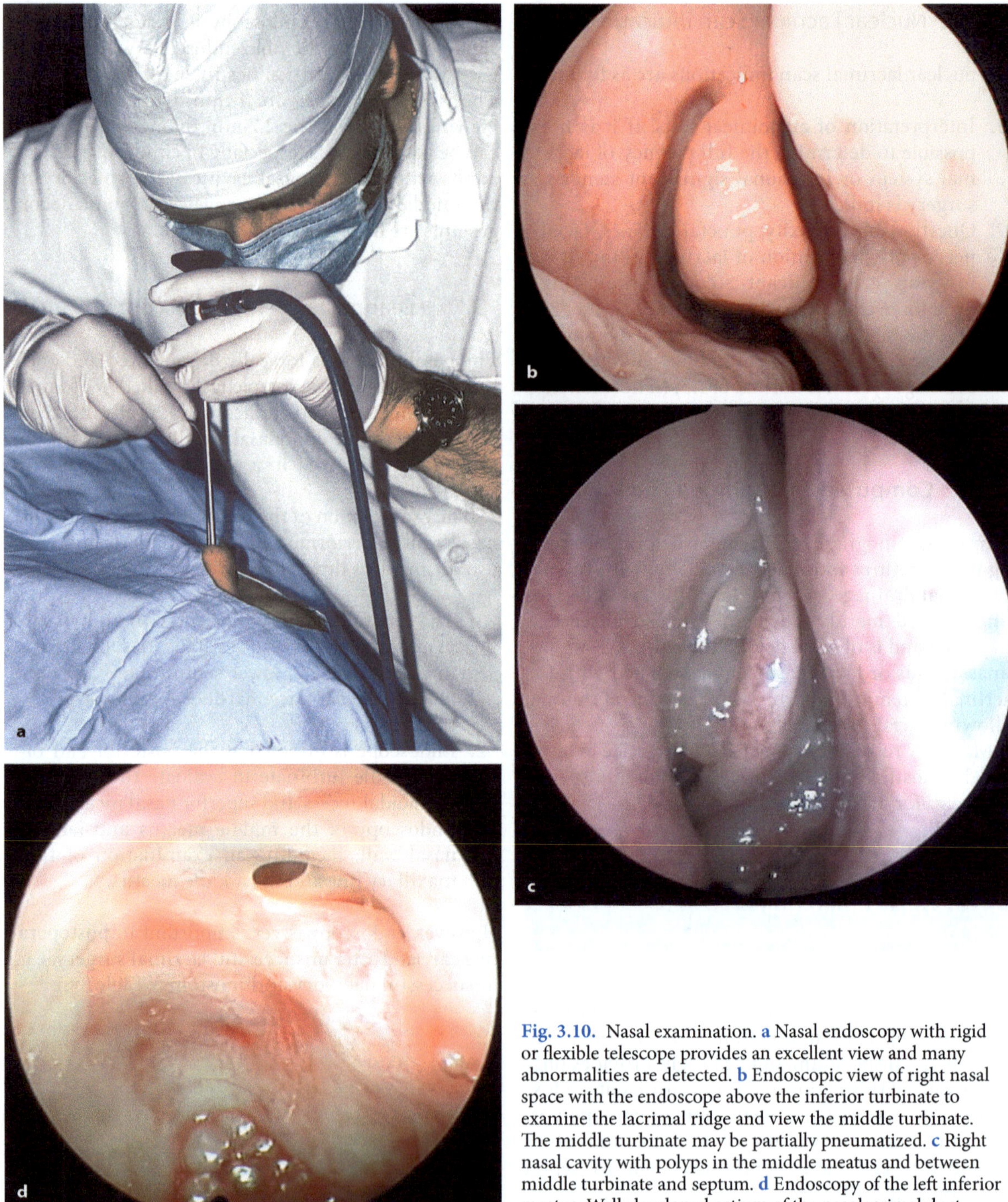

Fig. 3.10. Nasal examination. a Nasal endoscopy with rigid or flexible telescope provides an excellent view and many abnormalities are detected. b Endoscopic view of right nasal space with the endoscope above the inferior turbinate to examine the lacrimal ridge and view the middle turbinate. The middle turbinate may be partially pneumatized. c Right nasal cavity with polyps in the middle meatus and between middle turbinate and septum. d Endoscopy of the left inferior meatus. Well-developed ostium of the nasolacrimal duct

Table 3.6. Nasal endoscopy in lacrimal surgery

Preoperative examination	Assessment of anatomical abnormalities potentially affected proposed lacrimal surgery (nasal cavity extent, septal deviation, hypertrophic turbinate, mucosa appearance, previous nasal surgery)
	Assessment nasal pathology causing lacrimal symptoms (tumor, Wegener's granulomatosis, etc.)
	Observation of lacrimal transport (fluorescein)
Endonasal surgery	Lacrimal pathways intubation (turbinate infraction, dacryocystocoele incision, extraction of probes, etc.)
	Endonasal dacryocystorhinostomy (translumination, middle turbinate resection, septoplasty, bleeding control, laser EDCR, etc.)
	Conjunctivocystorhinostomy with primary EDCR (control tube position, turbinate resection, septoplasty, etc.)
Postoperative care	Endonasal follow-up post-endonasal and external lacrimal surgery (cleaning of the nasal cavity, size, and location of the DCR opening, Jones tube position, etc.
	Failed lacrimal surgery (to determine any compromise of the opening, to diagnose any lesions obstructing the opening such as granulomas, fibrous tissue, polyps, synechiae, etc.)
Revision lacrimal surgery	Revision DCR (middle turbinate resection, anterior ethmoidectomy, removing fibrous tissue, etc.)
	Conjunctivodacryocystorhinostomy (reinsertion and removing obstruction tissue)

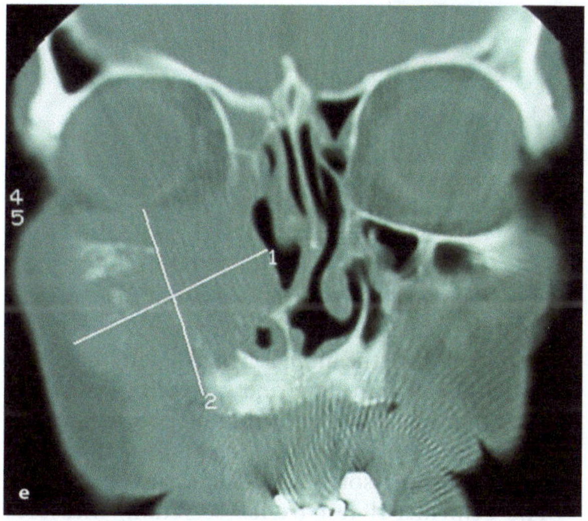

Fig. 3.10. (*Continued*) **e** Coronal CT scan of orbits and sinuses shows right maxillary sinus carcinoma with intraorbital growing. The patient was treated with a endonasal DCR for epifora and dacryocystitis. Suspected masses were found around the sac and spinocelullar carcinoma was histologically determined. (From [14])

3.8 Lacrimal System Endoscopy

3.8.1 Secretory Tests

If there is any suspicion of dry eye, the secretory tests should be done. A dry eye is usually suspected in the absence of any marginal tear strip, but the tear meniscus can be low or elevated if there is reflex tearing and/or if the tear film contains mucin, flakes, or filaments [20, 25].

Secretory tests include Schirmer's tests, bengal rose staining test, break-up test, and lysozyme lysis test (Table 3.7). These tests are helpful for the evaluation of tear production and indicate which component of the precorneal tear film is disturbed [11]. The treatment of a dry eye is quite different from anatomical or functional obstructions of the lacrimal system.

3.8.2 Schirmer's Tests

Quantification of tear production in the office setting is routinely done with Schirmer test strip.

Table 3.7. Evaluation of Schirmer tests

Test	Measured tear production	Normal
Schirmer I without anesthetic	Basic + reflex	10–35 (under 40 years, >15 mm; over 40 years, <10 mm
Schirmer I with anesthetic	Basic	Under 40 years, 10 mm; over 40 years, 5 mm
Schirmer II with anesthetic (trigeminal nerve stimulation)	Reflex	15 mm and more

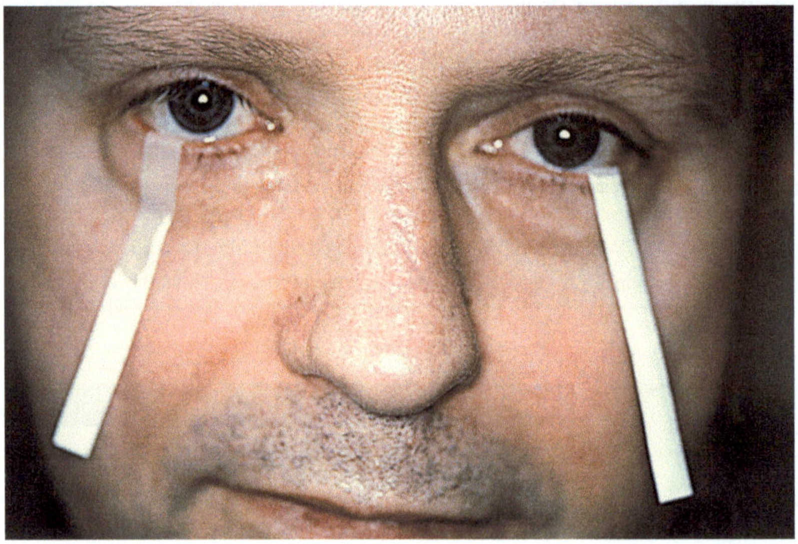

Fig. 3.11. Schirmers test

3.8.2.1 Performance

White Whatman filter paper in 35×5-mm strips is folded 5 mm from one end which is placed into the inferior fornix at the junction of the medial two-thirds and the other lateral one-third of the lower eyelid.

In semi-dardened room, the patient, without any eye drops, should not be stimulated verbally but is asked to blink normally for 5 min.

The amount of wetting to the paper is measured from the fold along its length after the paper has been removed.

There are distinguished tests with or without anesthetics.

Regarding performance, Schirmer I (basic + reflex secretion) is performed without any topical anesthetic (Table 3.6). Schirmer I with anesthetic (basic secretion test) is performed if a dry eye syndrome is suspected and the Schirmer's I is normal [9]. The principle of this test is in the elimination of the reflex contribution from the main lacrimal gland (including the irritation from the Schirmer test strips) with topical anesthetic instilled into the inferior formix [6]. The basic, non-reflex contribution of the tear production from the accessory glands is measured.

The Schirmer II test (reflex secretion) measures the reflex tearing derived from the main lacrimal gland. A topical anesthetic is applied to the eye to eliminate the reflex tearing from the local inflammation and irritation [6]. A trigeminal nerve is then stimulated either with a cotton applicator applied to the nasal mucosa or with ammonium chloride on a cotton pledget at the external nares. The amount of paper strip wetting is more than that elicited in the basic secretion test and represents the reflex secretion. This test is seldom used because the reflex secretion is usually intact [12] (Fig. 3.11).

3.8.2.2 Break-up Time

Break-up time indicates the function of the mucin layer or perhaps a reflex hypersecretion of an aqueous component of the tears. One drop of fluorescein is instilled into the external canthus of a lower lid and the patient is instructed to blink once and then to keep his eyes open. The holes developed in the tear film are observed at the cornea through a slit-lamp with illumination through the cobalt filter. The normal break-up time should be approximately 15–30 s. A break-up time of less than 10 s indicates a deficiency and the epiphora should be treated with libricating eye drops [9, 11].

3.8.2.3 Bengal Rose Staining

Bengal rose staining test is similar to a break-up time test. One drop of bengal rose is placed in the eye and the patient blinks several times for 1 min. Interpalpebral staining with bengal rose areas are then found in the dry eye. With both tests, staning of cornea is sought as lagophthalmos or incomplete blinking may exist, leading to reflex epiphora.

3.8.2.4 Lysozyme Lysis Test

The amount of a lysozyme activity and concentration is decreased in hypersecretion and in hyposecretion, and it usually precedes clinical symptoms. A lysozyme activity (and concentration) is estimated on the basis of the inhibition of the growth of the bacterium *Micrococcus lysodicticus*.

3.9 Conclusion

The purpose of the examination tests is to distinguish between epiphora and lacrimation, and between anatomic and physiological dysfunction. In most patients with epiphora the history, palpation and inspection, fluorescein dye disappearance test, diagnostic probing, and syringing are sufficient to determine drainage function, location, and extension of the anatomical block; if not, dacryocystography or nuclear scintigraphy can be helpful. In anatomical obstruction, it must be determined where the obstruction is located (presaccal, saccal, postsaccal) and the extent of an obstruction, if possible. Assessing canaliculi is essential. If the obstruction of one canaliculus is found, it is necessary to evaluate the other canaliculus. Once an anatomical obstruction in the lacrimal system has been located, the appropriate surgical procedure can then be chosen (Table 3.8). If surgical therapy is indicated, one should be able to say for whom the lid surgery may be more appropriate and for whom it may not.

However, it is important to bear in mind that with many diagnostic tests available to evaluate the patency of the lacrimal drainage system, there is no rigid unchanging standard approach to a patient with epiphora, and the treatment should not be decided without thorough consideration [28]. The recommended surgery can be influenced by the age of a patient, the previous therapy, history, motivation for surgical procedures, as well as other reasons.

Table 3.8. Management of lacrimal obstruction based on site of obstruction. *DCR* dacryocystorhinostomy, *CDCR* conjunctivodacryocystorhinostomy

Obstruction	Schema	Other factors	Recommended surgery
Saccal or subsaccal obstruction	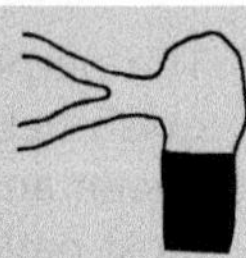		DCR
Canalicular stenosis	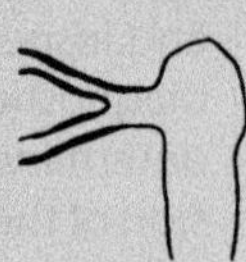		Intubation Laser canaliculoplasty + intubation DCR + intubation
Total common canalicular medial end obstruction	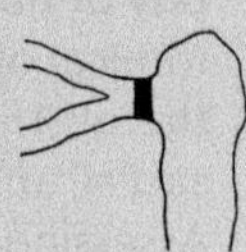		DCR with common internal puncto-plasty Laser dacryoplasty + intubation
Total common canalicular lateral end obstruction	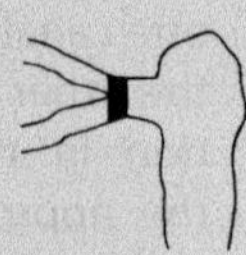		Canaliculodacryocystorhinostomy
Total individual canalicular obstruction, >8 mm from punctum	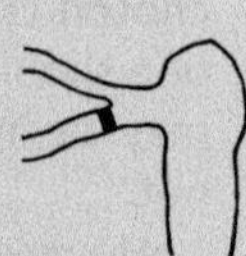	Opposite canaliculus patent	DCR
	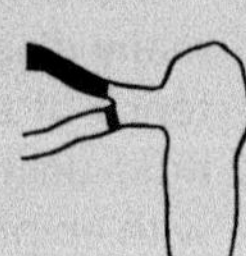	Opposite canaliculus obstructed	Canaliculodacryocystorhinostomy
Total individual canalicular obstruction, <8 mm from punctum	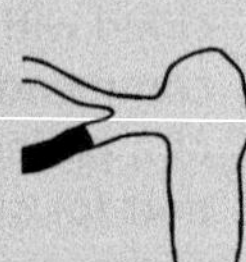	Opposite canaliculus patent	DCR
	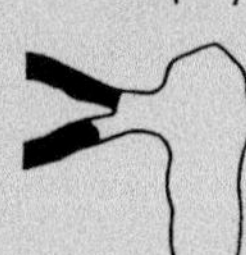	Opposite canaliculus obstructed	CDCR
Combined upper/lower canalicular obstruction	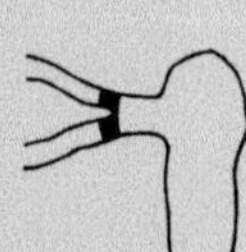	Either canaliculus patent >8 mm from punctum	Canaliculodacryocystorhinostomy
	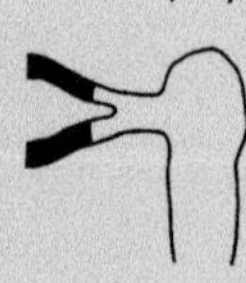	Neither canaliculus patent <8 mm from punctum	CDCR
Eyelid malposition, laxity			Lid surgery

References

1. Gonnering RS (1994) Dacryocystorhinostomy and conjunctivodacryocystorhinostomy. In: Dortzbach RK (ed) Ophthalmic plastic surgery: prevention and management of complications. Raven Press, New York, pp 237–250
2. Guzek JP et al. (1996) Lacrimal testing: the dye disappearance test and the Jones test. Ann Ophthalmol 28:357–363
3. Hagele E, Guzek JP, Shavlik GW (1994) Lacrimal testing. Ophthalmology 101:612–617
4. Hähnel S, Hansen O, Zake S et al. (1995) Der Wert der Spiral-CT zur Diagnose von Stenosen der ableitenden Tränenwege. Fortschr Roentgenstr 163:210–214
5. Hoffmann KT et al. (1999) High-resolution conjunctival contrast-enhanced MRI dacryocystography. Neuroradiography 41:208–213
6. Hornblass A, Herschorn BJ (1987) Lacrimal diagnosis. In: Smith BC (ed) Ophthalmic plastic and reconstructive surgery, vol 2. Mosby, St. Louis, pp 914–920
7. Hornblass A (1973) A simple taste test for lacrimal obstruction. Arch Ophthalmol 90:435–436
8. Hurwitz JJ, Welham RAN (1975) Radiography in functional lacrimal testing. Br J Ophthalmol 59:323–331
9. Hurwitz JJ (1996) The lacrimal system. Lippincott-Raven Publishers, Philadelphia
10. Hurwitz JJ, Molgat Y (1994) Nasolacrimal drainage system evaluation. Ophthalmol Clin N Am 7:393–406
11. Hurwitz JJ, Molgat Y (1993) Radiological test of lacrimal drainage. Diagnostic value versus cost-effectiveness. Lacrimal system. Symposium on the Lacrimal System, Brussels, 23–24 May, 1992, pp 15–26
12. Kanski JK (1999) Clinical ophthalmology. Butterworth-Heinemann, Oxford
13. Khan MS, Jones NS (2002) Endonasal (DCR) for the treatment of obstructive epiphora: otorhinolaryngologist, ophthalmologist or both? ENT News 11:55–59
14. Komínek P, Červenka S, Müllner K (2003) The lacrimal diseases. Diagnosis and treatment. Maxdorf, Prague
15. Lloyd GAS, Welham RAN (1974) Subtraction macrodacryocystography. Br J Radiol 47:379–382
16. Mannor GE, Millman AL (1991) The prognostic value of preoperative dacryocystography in endoscopic intranasal dacrocystorhinostomy. Am J Ophthalmol 113:134–137
17. MacEwen CJ, Young JDH (1991) The fluorescein disappearance test: an evaluation of its use in infants. J Pediatr Ophthalmol Strab 28:302–305
18. Meyer DR, Antonello A, Linberg JV (1990) Assessment of tear drainage after canalicular obstruction using fluorescein dye disappearance. Ophthalmology 97:370–374
19. Müllner K, Bodner E, Mannor GE (1999) Endoscopy of the lacrimal system. Br J Ophthalmol 83:949–952
20. Olver J (2002) Colour atlas of lacrimal surgery. Butterworth-Heinemann, Oxford
21. Patrinely JR, Anderson RL (1986) A review of lacrimal drainage surgery. Ophthalmol Plast Reconstr Surg 2:97–102
22. Sahlin S, Chen E (1996) Evaluation of the lacrimal drainage function by the drop test. Am J Ophthalmol 122:701–708
23. Walther EK, Köster O, Straehler-Pohl HJ (1989) Dakryozystographie in digilater Subtraktionstechnik. Laryngol Rhinol Otol 68:396–400
24. Walther EK (1991) Digitale Subtraktionsdakryozystographie bei obstruktiven Tränenwegserkrankungen und ihrer operativen Behandlung nach Veis-Claus. Otorinolaryngol Nova 1:233–241
25. Waltz KL, Nesi FA, Gladstone GJ (1994) Epiphora. In: Margo CE (ed) Diagnostic problems in clinical ophthalmology. Saunders, Philadelphia, pp 115–118
26. Watkins LM, Janfaza P, Tubin PA (2003) The evolution of endonasal dacryocystorhinostomy. Surv Ophthalmol 48:73–84
27. Welham RAN (1998) Investigations for patients undegoing lacrimal surgery. Eye 12:334–336
28. Yeatts RP (2000) Acquired nasolacrimal duct obstruction. Oculoplast Surg 13:719–729
29. Zappia RH, Milder B (1972) Lacrimal drainage function: the Jones fluorescein test. Am J Ophthalmol 74:154–159
30. Zappia RH, Milder B (1972) Lacrimal drainage function: the fluorescein dye disappearance test. Am J Ophthalmol 74:160–162

Chapter 4

Nasolacrimal Probing and Intubation

4

Lisa Pierroth, D.A. Della Rocca and R.C. Della Rocca

Core Messages

- We perform the probing first through the upper canaliculus and then through the inferior canaliculus.
- It is important to not rotate the punctual dilator horizontally before 2 mm of vertical dilation, so as to avoid damage to the vertical part of the canaliculus.
- The probe is advanced medially until a hard stop is felt. The lid is pulled laterally to ensure that the horizontal canaliculus is not kinked, as false passageways must be avoided.
- The probe is passed 18–20 mm in children before entering the nose through the obstructed site typically at the valve of Hasner.
- The Crawford retrieval hook is placed perpendicular to the operating room table towards the inferior turbinate while hugging the lateral wall. Be sure you know where the open face of the hook is facing.

Contents

4.1 Introduction and Background of the Technique

Congenital nasolacrimal duct obstruction is the most common cause for epiphora in the newborn. The most common location of obstruction is at the opening of the nasolacrimal system due to an imperforate valve of Hasner [1]. Other causes of obstruction may be atypical in the nasolacrimal duct to end, within the bony nasal lacrimal canal, in the wall of the maxillary sinus, or below the inferior turbinate. The nasolacrimal canal may end as a tube of mucosa lateral to the inferior turbinate.

Embryologically, the lacrimal system proceeds from proximal to distal and 30% of full-term newborns present with an imperforate valve of Hasner [2]. Most infants undergo spontaneous valve opening by age 6 weeks, but the remaining 10% may require probing of the nasolacrimal system. The length of the nasolacrimal excretory system is 22–24 mm in the 1-year-old child.

Chronic epiphora must be carefully evaluated to rule out other causes of lacrimation such as conjunctivitis, punctual occlusion, canalicular stenosis, amniotocele, dacryoocystocele, epiblepharon, entropion, or ectropion. Congenital glaucoma is usually associated with photophobia and excess lacrimation.

An amniotocele, which is uncommon, is caused by amniotic fluid and conjunctival fluid trapped between the common internal punctae (valve of Rosenmüller) and the valve of Hasner, and it presents as a bluish fluctuant mass in the medial canthal region and should be differentiated from a meningo(encephaolo)cele or a capillary hemangioma.

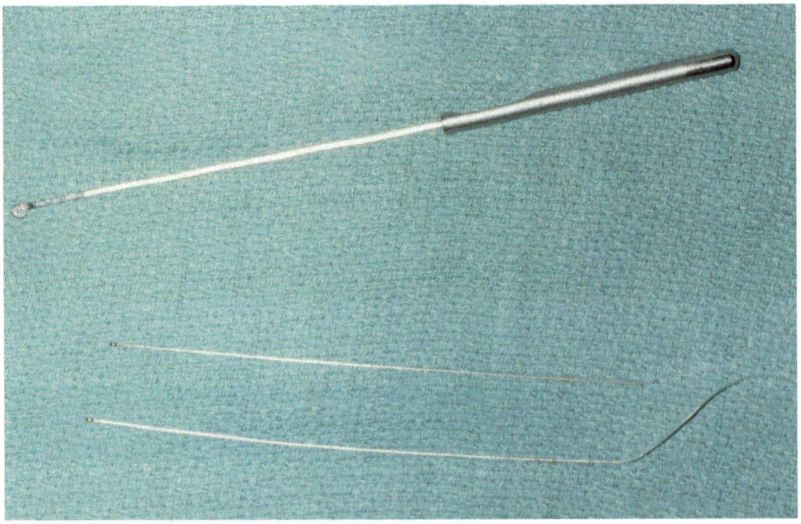

Fig. 4.1. Crawford tubes (JedMed) and preferred retrieval hook: set 28-0185

4.2 Indications and Contraindications

Gentle inferior massage over the area of the nasolacrimal sac and lacrimal crest for infants with chronic and persistent tearing and or mild to moderate mucopurulent discharge due to nasolacrimal obstruction. Nasolacrimal massage may help to treat the obstruction in the infant and reduce the risk of subsequent dacryocystitis. Concurrently, we recommend a 10-day cause of topical antibiotic drops. Obtain a culture and sensitivity of the discharge if possible to define the antibiotic sensitivity. Systemic antibiotics are required if signs of subacute or acute dacryocystitis exists.

If conservative treatment does not relieve symptoms of tearing due to nasolacrimal obstruction, probing may be indicated between 6 and 13 months of age [3]. The failure rate of initial probing significantly increases after 13 months of age, as does the number and complexity of subsequent procedures that may be required to repair the problem. With persistent mucopurulent discharge, probing is done earlier, perhaps at age 6 months or before depending on the severity of dacryocystitis. Newborns presenting with an amniotocele usually require probing within 10 days of diagnosis.

If probing fails (as it does in approximately 10% of cases), the insertion of a silastic intubation tube is advised with subsequent probing. Likewise, a silastic intubation tube is used if probing is not achieved easily because of a tightened nasolacrimal pathway. In our experience it is likely that silastic intubation is required initially at 15 months of age or older. Persistent tearing and/or dacryocystitis, despite multiple probings and intubation, is an indication for dacryocystorhinostomy at 2 years or older (see Chap. 5).

4.3 Instrumentation

Lacrimal probing instruments include a punctual dilator, Bowman probes, lacrimal irrigation cannula, irrigation tip, BSS-filled syringe, lacrimal intubation system (Crawford silicone stent set 28-0185, JedMed Instrument Company, St. Louis, Mo.) and a retrieval hook to Silastic intubation tube (supplied with the lacrimal intubation set; Fig. 4.1).

4.4 Anesthesia

We recommend general endotracheal anesthesia for children during nasolacrimal probing. Mask anesthesia can be used when the silastic tube is removed.

4.5 Operative Technique

After induction of general anesthesia, neurosurgical cottonoids moistened with oxymetazoline hydrochloride 0.05% (Afrin spray) are placed medial and lateral to the inferior turbinate for vasoconstriction to im-

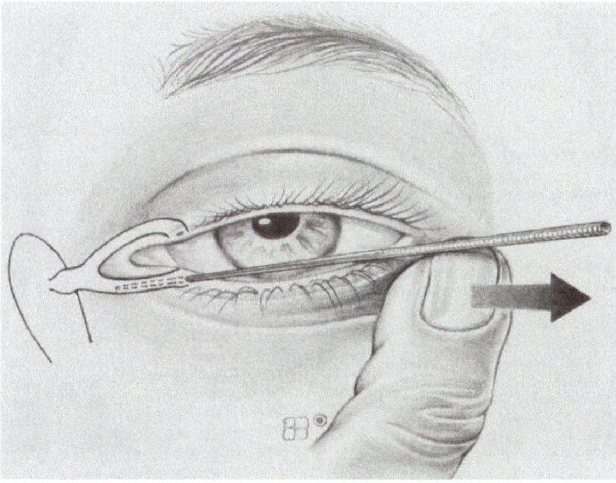

Fig. 4.2. The punctal dilator is used to dilate the inferior punctum, and then the superior punctum

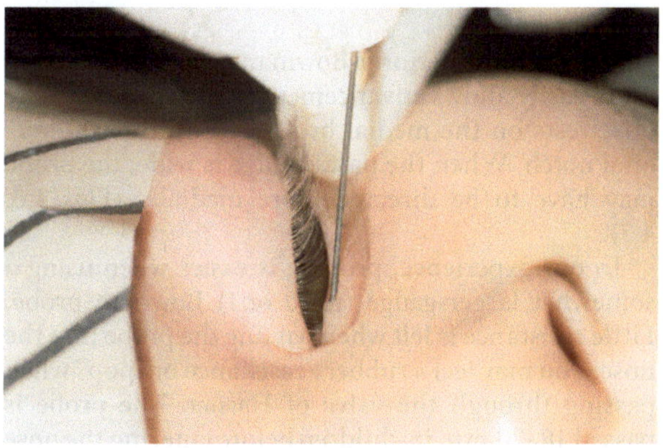

Fig. 4.3. Bowman probe 0 or 00 is passed horizontally with lateral lower eyelid traction until the bone is palpated with the probe

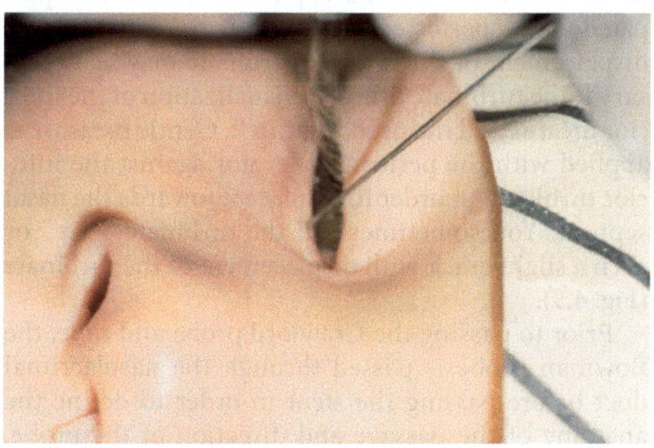

Fig. 4.4. Same as Fig. 4.3

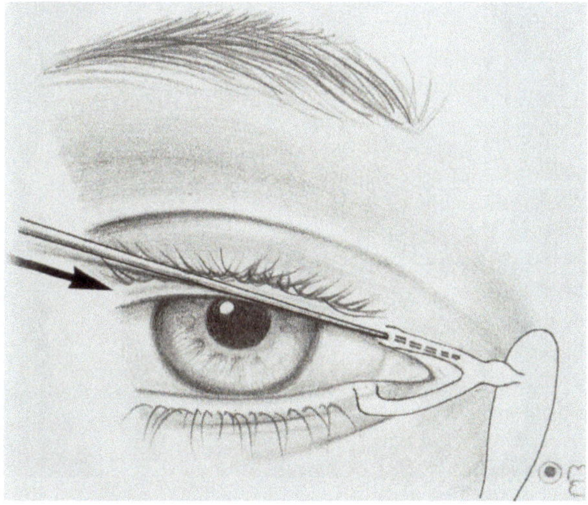

Fig. 4.5. The upper canaliculus is kinked by the lacrimal probe. Avoid this by placing the upper lid on lateral traction as the probe is advanced

prove visualization as well as decrease bleeding. Fiber-optic headlight is used to aid visualization of the nose. Baynonette forceps are used to position cottonoids beneath and medial to the inferior turbinate. The cottonoids are removed after 5–10 min.

We perform the probing first through the upper canaliculus and then through the inferior canaliculus.

The length of the Bowman probe is measured prior to using the dilator in order to assess length of passage through the nasolacrimal canal or nose, repectively. The upper canaliculus is dilated carefully with a blunt punctual dilator for a distance of 2 mm. The punctual dilator is now rotated horizontally and parallel to the superior horizontal canaliculus. It is important to not rotate the punctual dilator horizontally before 2 mm of vertical dilation so as to avoid damage to the vertical part of the canaliculus.The punctal dilator is withdrawn and a no. 0 or 1 Bowman probe is passed immediately after withdrawal of the punctual dilator vertically for 2 mm and then reoriented horizontally. The same gentle lateral lid retraction will decrease the risk of false passageway (Figs. 4.2–4.4).

The probe is advanced medially until a hard stop is felt. The lid is pulled laterally to ensure that the horizontal canaliculus is not kinked as false passageways must be avoided (Fig. 4.5).

The Bowman probe is then gently rotated vertically within the bony nasolacrimal canal while hug-

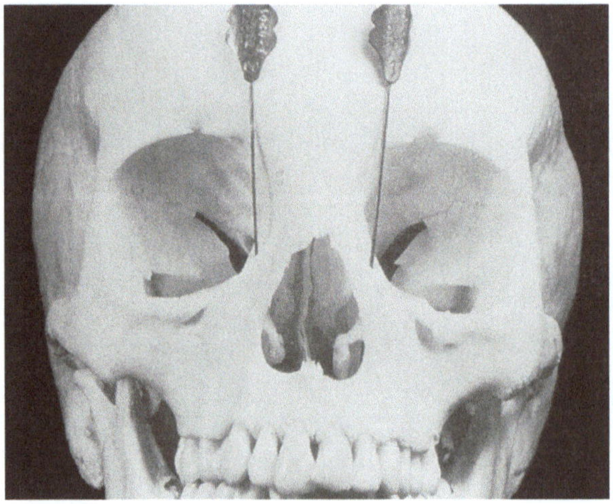

Fig. 4.6. In skull with typical nasal bridge, probe at brow will be directed at 10–15° angles from a superior to inferior direction

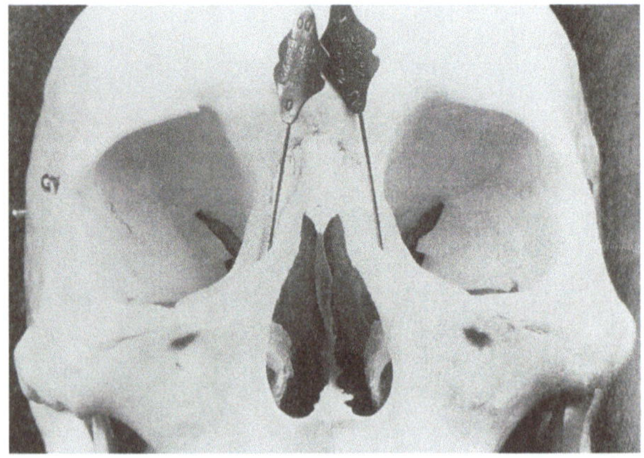

Fig. 4.7. Broadened nasal bridge probe direction will be parallel to each other as probe passes through nasolacrimal ducts

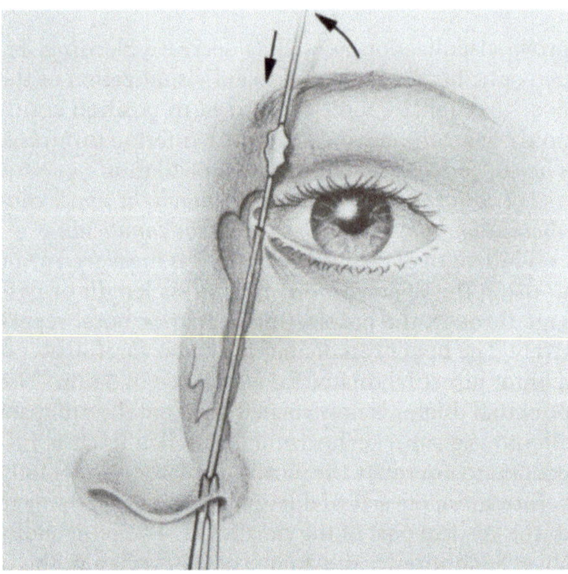

Fig. 4.8. Note inferomedial direction of Bowman probe as it passes through the canaliculus, lacrimal sac, nasolacrimal duct and the valve of Hasner

ging the brow superiorly. Bowman probe position that more easily allows advancement of the probe into the nose rests on the medial brow close to the supraorbital notch. When the nasal bridge is wide, the probe may have to be directed more medially (Figs. 4.6, 4.7).

In our experience, probing is easier when using a somewhat larger-gauge (no. 0 or 1) Bowman probe. Little resistance is felt when passing the probe into the nose. You may feel a rubbery resistance or "pop" when passing through the valve of Hasner. The probe is passed 18–20 mm in children before entering the nose through the obstructed site typically at the valve of Hasner (Fig. 4.8).

The probe may be identified 20 mm into the nares either by direct or endoscopic visualization or palpated with a periosteal elevator. Medial infracture or displacement of the inferior turbinate may be necessary if the turbinate prevents visualization of the inferior meatus and the probe within it. Gentle pressure is applied with the periosteal elevator against the inferior turbinate in order to displace it towards the nasal septum. You sometimes feel the turbinate "give" or even a slight crack with displacement of the turbinate (Fig. 4.9).

Prior to passing the Crawford probe and tube, the Bowman probe is passed through the nasolacrimal duct before passing the stent in order to define the anatomy of the passage and direction of the probe.

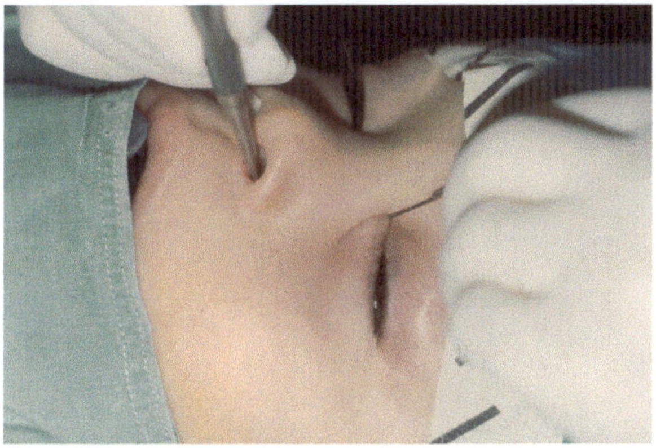

Fig. 4.9. Freer elevator is used to displace the inferior turbinate medially to facilitate passage of Bowman probe when resistance is encountered. Some nasal bleeding may develop with this maneuver. Pediatric merocel packing is useful in stopping the bleeding

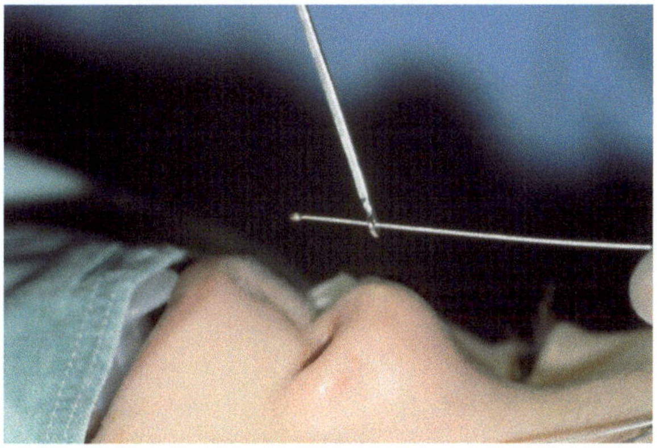

Fig. 4.10. A retrieval hook grasping the Crawford probe with tube externally

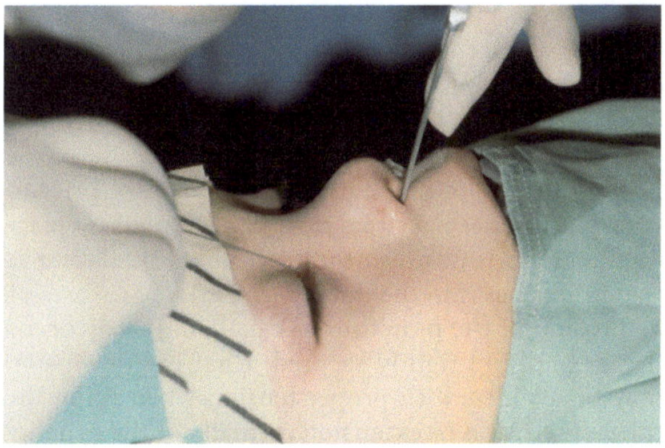

Fig. 4.11. With Crawford tube passed into the nose, and manipulated superiorly, the retrieval hook is passed into the inferior meatus to grasp the olive tip of the probe. When grasped, the metal probe is pulled in a superior direction from above to fortify the grasp, and the probe is then pulled out of the nose in a slightly medial direction

This will define the length of the tube required to the probe through the ostium of the duct and into the nares The Crawford metal probes are thinner and more difficult to pass than the firm Bowman probe.

The olive tips are placed first through the upper canalicular and nasolacrimal duct, and then the lower canaliculus.

They may be received with the Crawford hook (C106 from Roger Klein, Palmer Puerto Rico) or a small hemostat. The Crawford retrieval hook is placed perpendicular to the operating room table towards the inferior turbinate while hugging the lateral wall. Be sure you know where the open face of the hook is facing. The stent is palpated with the Crawford hook or freer elevator. The hook is advanced a few millimeters with the eye of the hook facing laterally. The olive tip of the probe is palpated, hooked, and advanced out the nose as the Crawford probe is gently pushed from above. Limit grasping the nasal mucosa with the hook (Figs. 4.10, 4.11).

Once both stents have been passed into the nose, proper positioning of the loop of silastic tubing within the eye should be evaluated in the eye. The metallic probes are pulled off or cut off. The loose tubing is pulled anteriorly using needle holders and, following a single tie to allow the tubes to retract 15 mm into the nose, four more knots are completed preferably tying the knots over a no. 1 Bowman probe. The tied tubes are then allowed to retract into the nose. Observe for intranasal bleeding at this time. Prior to extubation, if bleeding is noted, gently pack the nose with a narrow merocel dampened with xylocaine and epinephrine (Fig. 4.12).

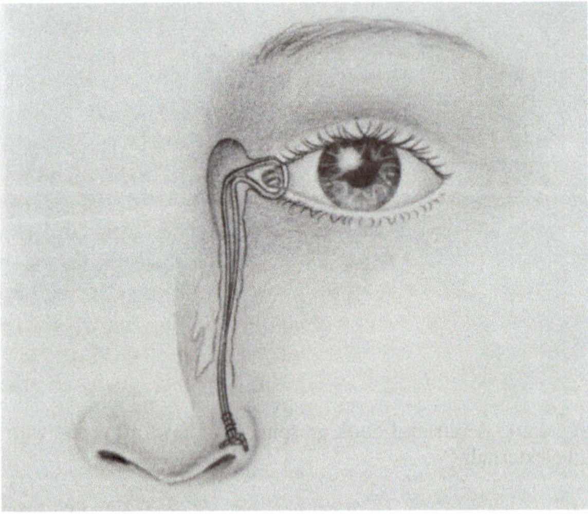

Fig. 4.12. Silastic tube ends are tied with five single knots and allowed to retract 15 mm into the nose

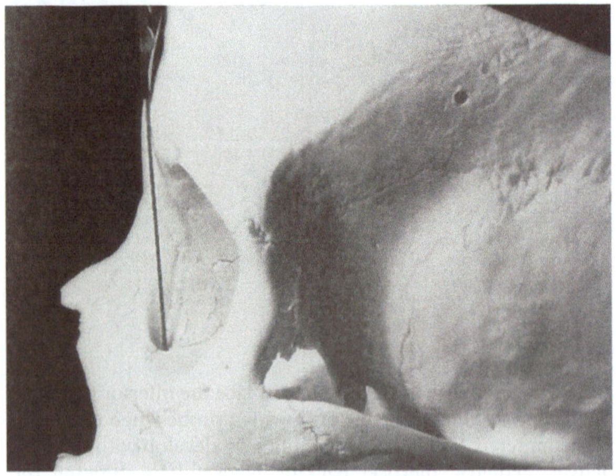

Fig. 4.13. With Bowman probe in place the finger is placed over the anterior lacrimal crest to help direct the probe into the duct. This obviates the creation of false passages

4.6 Postoperative Care and Complications

Topical combined antibiotic and steroid ointment (e.g., Tobradex) is to be used four times daily for a period of 1 week after nasolacrimal duct probing or intubation. Systemic antibiotics, preferably Amoxacillin, is used for 3–4 days postoperatively. If some persistence of intranasal bleeding exists and prior to extubation use, merocel to pack the nose dampened with osymetazoline hydrochloride 0.05% (Afrin) or xylocaine 1% with 1:100,000 epinephrine solution is used. Await for bleeding to subside and in most instances the packing can be removed prior to extubaion. The child can usually be discharged several hours after completion of the procedure in an ambulatory setting. Significant epiphora and chronic dacryocystitis with mucous discharge in a child 6–13 months of age can usually be treated successfully with nasolacrimal probing alone. Nasolacrimal probing done after 15 months of age or older requires the use of silastic intubation. Good correlation of surgical anatomy, planning, and appropriate timing of the procedure increases the success rate and decreases the possibility of complications. The silastic tube is left in place for 4–6 months, if possible. Early on, it is advisable to place and tape at periphery of perforated protective shield over the eye with sufficient openings for the child to see out of the eye.

Bloody tears or bloody discharge from the nose can be expected up to 2 weeks after probing and need no further treatment unless more than a few drops.

The surgical pitfall of displacing the probe prior to entering the nasolacrimal duct is prevented by placing the index finger over the anterior lacrimal crest as the probe goes into the duct (Fig. 4.13).

Erosion of the punctum or canaliculus may occur if tubes are too tightly secured. Chaffing or erosion may be avoided with proper tension when tying the tubes. If erosion or extension medially of the canaliculus has occurred, the tubes need to be removed and the erosion will suitably heal.

Prolapse of the nasolacrimal tubing may occur because the child rubs the eye too vigorously. It is advisable to inform the family of the child of this possibility to limit their concern if it occurs. Tube prolapse can be avoided by having the child wear an eye shield early after probing which can be kept in place at bedtime for several weeks. Tube reposition can be achieved with a bayonette forceps and a headlight or nasal endoscope for visualization with mask anesthesia. Less frequently, the tube is removed. Strong effort to reposition is particularly important during the first month after placement.

Granulomas may occur at the punctum which need to be excised. We recommend removal of the tubing system at the same time. If granuloma is small, allow the tube to remain in place for as long as possible.

4.7 Tube Removal

Generally, the tube is left in place for at least 6 months after intubation and once symptoms are stable [4]. If there is unroofing or stretching of the canaliculus, earlier removal may be considered.

After 3–6 months, the tube can be removed . It can sometimes be done in the office but in most instances requires mask anesthesia in the operating room. In the office, a drop of anesthetic is applied to the fornix. Similarly, in the office or with mask anesthesia, the tube is grasped superiorly and transected. The tube is then retrieved through the superior canaliculus. When the tube is attached to the septum it may be difficult to remove the tube through the canaliculus. An antibiotic/steroid eye drop four times daily is recommended for 10 days after removal of the tube.

Reference

1. Crawford JS: Intubation of obstructions in the lacrimal system. Can J Ophthalmol 1977;12:289–292
2. Bedrossian EJ Jr: The lacrimal system. In: Tasman W, Jaeger E (eds) Duane's foundation of clinical ophthalmology, vol 1, 1996; 30:179–187
3. Katowitz JA, Welsh MG: Timing of initial probing and irrigation in congenital nasolacrimal duct obstruction. Ophthalmology 1987; 94:698–704
4. Welsh MG, Katowitz JA: Timing of silastic tubing removal after intubation for congenital nasolacrimal duct obstruction. Ophthalmol Plast Reconstr Surg 1989; 5:43–48

Suggested Reading:

Lemke BN, Della Rocca RC: Surgery of the eyelids and orbit: an anatomical approach. East Norwalk, CT: Appleton and Lange, 1990. (Available through McGraw-Hill)

Della Rocca RC, Bedrossian EH, Arthurs BP: Ophthalmic plastic surgery: Decision making and techniques. New York: McGraw-Hill, 2003: 165–179, 181–187

Chapter 5

Dacryocystorhinostomy Surgical Technique

5

Manuel Bernal-Sprekelsen, Isam Alobid, Manuel Tomás-Barberán, R.C. Della Rocca and S.D. Schaefer

Core Messages

- Identification of the "maxillary line" prevents going too far posteriorly.
- The probing of the pathways is therefore essential to distinguish between a presaccal and a saccal/postsaccal obstruction.
- The inferiorly based mucosal flap, once put back in position, reduces the time of wound healing considerably.
- It is recommended to create a large dacryocystorhinostomy.
- Opening of the lacrimal sac should be in its superior third, facing the common canaliculus.
- Probing both canaliculi does not improve the result, but is helpful during the follow-up.
- Silicone probing remains in place for 2–3 weeks only.

Contents

5.1 Introduction

The search for an alternative to the external approach is motivated by the desire to improve the DCR success rate and to add other advantages, such as a better aesthetic result or better compliance by the patient. The endonasal DCR is a one-stage procedure that permits correction of associated pathology, such as septal deviation or chronic paranasal sinusitis, that may be a causative factor in lacrimal obstruction [1].

A first description of the feasibility of this approach was presented in a cadaver study by Rice [1], and the results on the first four patients published by McDonough and Meiring [2]. The rationale for endonasal approaches lies in the anatomy of the lacrimal pathways: about 80% are in the nose. An external scar (Fig. 5.1) is avoided, which leads to a better acceptance by the patients, mainly women. Functional results are at least as good as after external Toti procedures.

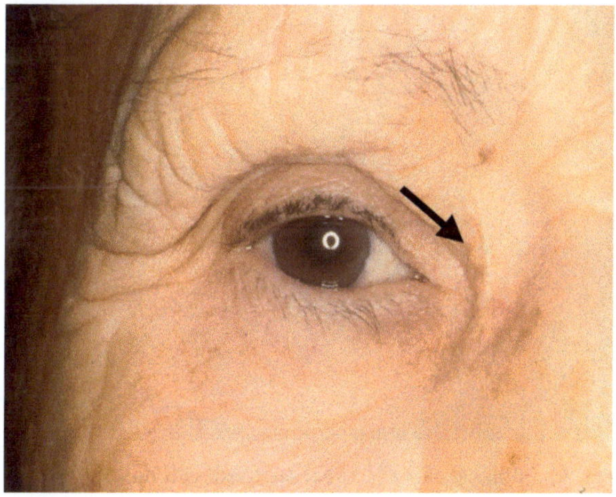

Fig. 5.1. Scar after external DCR

Acute infections, such as purulent dacryocystitis with or without involvement of the outer skin, are no formal contraindication as pus is drained into a contaminated nasal fossa. This may reduce the risk of angular vein thrombosis and intracranial extension of the infection through the ophthalmic vein into the cavernous sinus.

5.2 Indications and Contraindications

There are mainly four well-established indications for a DCR: epiphora, (relapsing) dacryocystitis, dacryocele, and dacryolithiasis, the latter being quite rare in our series. Whereas dacryocystitis is an easy indication (a simple inspection or palpation of the bulging sac (Fig. 5.2) may confirm it), chronic epiphora needs a differential diagnosis. Here, basically it is necessary to differentiate between a presaccal obstruction (in the punctum lacrimale, the superior or inferior canaliculus, or the common canaliculus) and an obstruction in the lacrimal sac or the nasolacrimal duct (saccal or postsaccal problem). Irrigation with saline solution or fluorescein dye application can also help to assess the patency of the pathways. On the contrary, dacryocystographies and CAT scans are not performed on a routine basis.

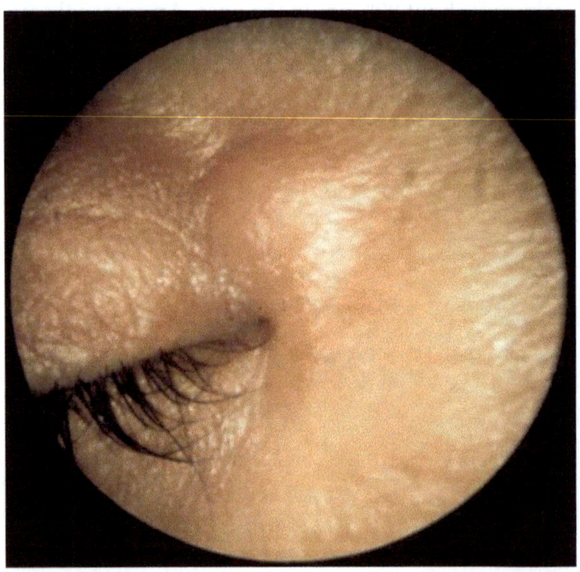

Fig. 5.2. Bulging of the lacrimal sac filled with mucous or pus. Smooth palpation may lead to evacuation through the punctum lacrimale

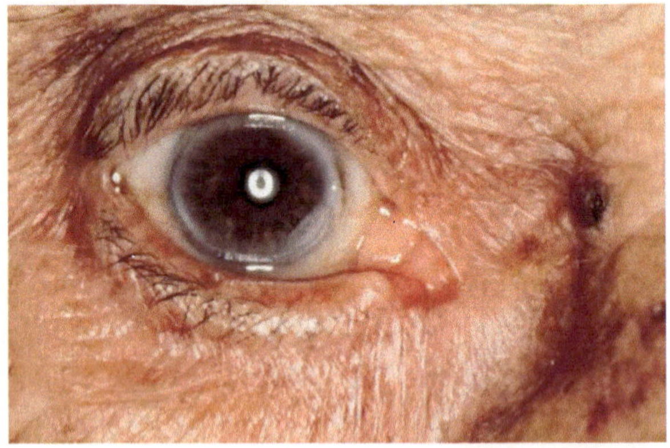

Fig. 5.3. Lagophthalmus as seen in elderly patients, as well as facial palsy, may lead to chronic epiphora

Clinical inspection should also assess the contact between the inferior lacrimal punctum and the conjunctiva. In patients with facial palsy lagophthalmus leads to epiphora and ectropion of the inferior eyelid in elderly persons impedes normal drainage of tears mimicking chronic epiphora also (Fig. 5.3).

5.3 Case History

A 22-year-old girl had recurrent dacyocystitis of the left side for 14 months. During the last episode the skin was involved by the infection and pus drained through a cutaneous fistula. Oral antibiotic treatment associated with eye drops containing steroids and antibiotic helped in reducing the infection. Figure 5.4 shows the residual state prior to DCR, which was performed endoscopically under general anesthesia. No further dacryocystitis occurred during a 4-year follow-up period.

5.4 Surgical Technique

Surgery was performed under general anesthesia [3–5]. Procedures under local anesthesia only are feasible in those cases when general anesthesia is not recommended or the patient preferred local anesthesia. Surgery under general anesthesia includes topical anesthesia of the nasal fossa, performed with neurosurgical cottonoids soaked in topical anesthetic and adrenaline (1:100,000), applied 10–15 min prior to surgery in order to achieve a good vasoconstriction.

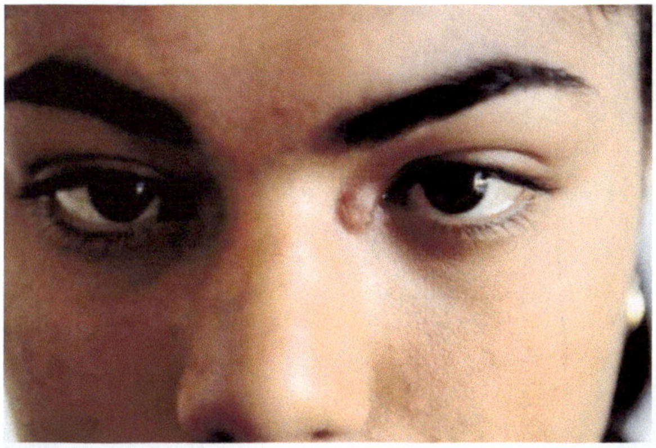

Fig. 5.4. Situation after an acute, purulent dacryocystitis with remnant scar in a young patient

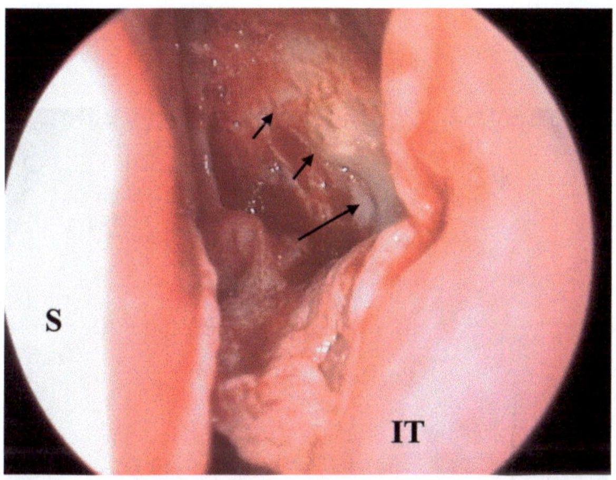

Fig. 5.5. Left nose. Exposure of the Agger nasi after elevation of the inferiorly based mucosal flap. *Small arrows* indicate the superior aspect of the "maxillary line," *large arrow* the partial exposure of the lacrimal sac after circumscribed drilling of the bone. *S* septum, *IT* inferior turbinate

For surgery under local anesthesia an intravenous sedation is performed. Additionally, to this and the topical anesthesia, infiltrations of the supratrochlear and infraorbital nerves (approximately 2 ml of bupivacain) are applied; however, topical anesthesia of the lacrimal sac itself may be difficult when an acute infection is present. Surgery is performed with a 30° or 45° rigid endoscope (Storz Company). The microscope might be suitable as well.

Occasionally, the head of the middle turbinate needs to be trimmed in order to achieve a proper approach to the lacrimal sac. Septal deviations facing the *Agger nasi* should be corrected prior to the DCR. If this is the only affected area, we then prefer a "mini-septoplasty" through an "L"-shaped mucosal incision, followed by circumscribed cartilage resection or correction and reposition of the mucosal flap. Providing a larger space between septum and lacrimal sac, the immediate post-operative care is easier to be carried out.

On the *Agger nasi*, two vertical incisions are made through the mucosa down to the bone. The posterior incision is placed vertically on the posterior edge of the *Crista maxillaris*, called the "maxillary line," in front of the uncinate process. The anterior incision is performed slightly anteriorly and superiorly to the middle turbinate, with a width of little more than 1 cm from the "maxillary line"; thus, an inferiorly based, mucoperiosteal flap is created on the *Agger nasi* and pushed towards the inferior turbinate (Fig. 5.5). Instruments like the Freer elevator (Karl Storz Company) or the bent Montserrat knife are useful for achieving a sharp dissection posteriorly (in front of the uncinate process), and to make a thorough subperiosteal dissection. Prior infiltration of this mucosa with local anesthesia and epinephrine (1:100,000) may be useful, but it is not done routinely. The flap measures about 1.5 cm in height and 1 cm in width. At the end of the DCR, this mucosal flap is repositioned, partially covering the lateral wall. Trimming of the flap may sometimes be necessary in order to prevent covering the new drainage of the lacrimal sac, but generally, the mucosa suffers a minor retraction, leaving the new ostium open once the flap is put back in its original position.

When the endoscopic approach was started, the mucosal flap created on the *Agger nasi* was resected in order to gain access to the ascending crista of the maxilla. This led to major formation of crusts, blood clots, and a long healing process, but also to a higher rate of cheek ecchymosis or emphysemas. During the past 5–6 years, the study incorporated a suggestion made by Massegur that was published recently [6], to preserve an inferiorly based mucosal flap on the *Agger nasi*, which then is replaced after the saccotomy, reducing considerably the period of scarring and preventing ecchymosis.

The "maxillary line" (Fig. 5.5) provides a clear anatomic landmark: the bone resection is performed from this edge anteriorly. The bone of this ascending process may be very strong. The true lacrimal bone,

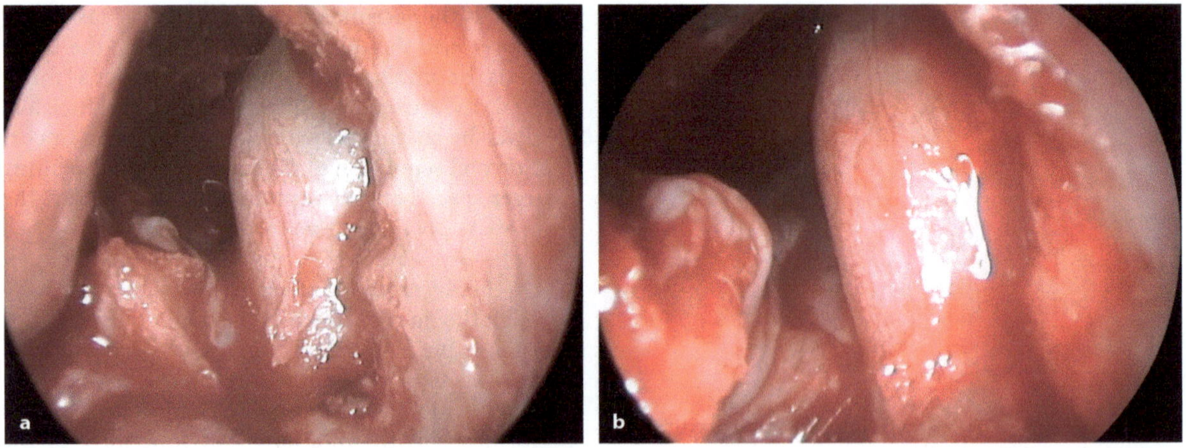

Fig. 5.6 a,b. Progressive removal of the *Processus ossis maxillaris* with the 90° Kerrisson rongeur until complete exposure of the sac. Pressure is applied from outside to produce a bulging

located more laterally and posteriorly, is quite thin and more fragile; thus, cold light fibers introduced through the inferior canaliculus provide a transillumination that shows where the bone usually is thinner, i.e., at the most posterior edge. Entering the lacrimal sac at the posterior aspect, where the contact with the periorbit might be very tight, and absence of bony separation between the lacrimal sac and the periorbit, which has been observed in about 10–15% of the cases, may cause a lesion to the periorbit with exposure of the orbital fat and bleeding into the orbit.

Dissection of the lacrimal sac can be achieved by means of different methods. Bone removal with the help of hammer and chisel, the latter directed towards the orbit, implies a strong confidence in the person holding the hammer. Backbiting of the process with Kerrison rongeurs, positioned at the very edge of the "maxillary line," are feasible as long as the bone is not too thick. In these cases we prefer to employ an ear-cutting burr under irrigation with saline to drill the ascending process of the maxilla, until a circumscribed exposure of the lacrimal sac surface is achieved (Fig. 5.6). The use of a diamond burr is recommended when the surgeon has less experience with this procedure. Care has to be taken to avoid the inferiorly based mucosal flap to become wrapped around the burr. If there is any doubt about the correct identification of the lacrimal sac, the surgeon can palpate the sac from outside or introduce a lacrimal probe through the inferior canaliculus and then push gently. The lacrimal sac

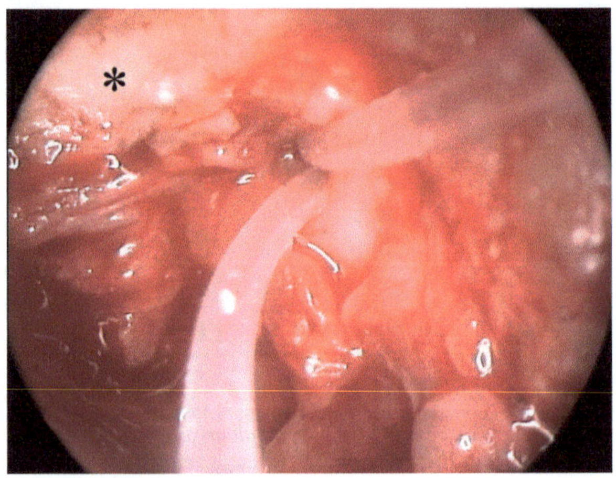

Fig. 5.7. Both ends of the silicone stent leaving the common canaliculus. *Asterisk* indicates remnant bone of the superior aspect of the *Processus ossis maxillaris*

may be identified by its bulging. Then, a 90° Kerrison rongeur is used to remove additional bone anteriorly and a 45° Kerrison rongeur to remove the bone superiorly until the entire medial wall and most of the anterior wall of the lacrimal sac is exposed in its superior aspect, where the common canaliculus enters the sac.

While a helping hand exercises a firm pressure from outside (best: putting a finger on the inner edge of the eye) a vertical incision is then made in the anterior face of the lacrimal sac with the help of a number

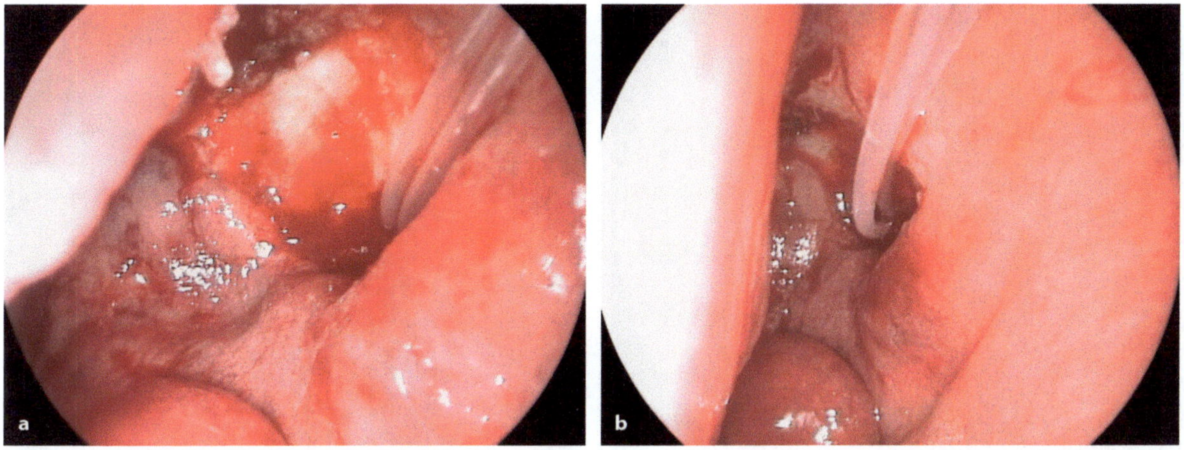

Fig. 5.8. Reposition of the mucosal flap. Note that the flap does not cover the silicone probe. Minor shrinking of the mucosal flap occurs; thus, not all parts of bone remain covered. The view provides an impression of the anatomical landmarks, the opening of the sac being above the head of the middle turbinate

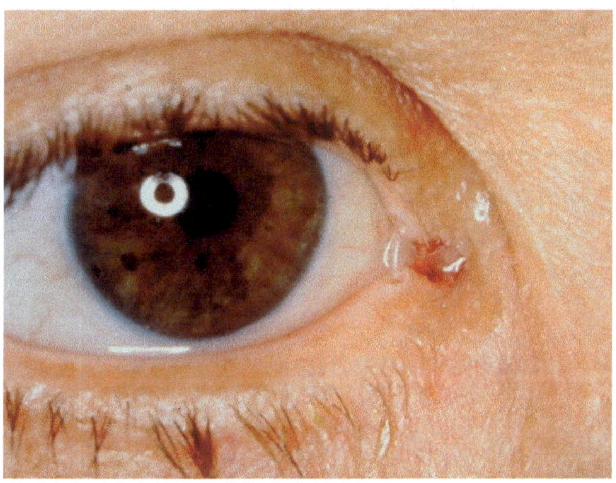

Fig. 5.9. Fixing of the silicone probe on the external nose should not impede opening of the eyelids

11 or a phaco knife. The pressure from outside prevents the sac to displace laterally when trying to make the incision. At this point, pus or mucus usually flows from the sac. The entire medial wall is removed using straight Blakesley forceps or true cutting forceps. In cases of severe inflammation or infection the medial wall is easily removed by sheer forces with the instrument. When inflamed or infected, the walls of the lacrimal sac become thick; thus, its incision may sometimes be too superficial.

The patency of the DCR is checked by a lacrimal probe passed into the nose via the inferior canaliculus, which is seen in the nasal fossa. Probing both canaliculi with a silicone catheter is used as a stent for 2–3 weeks after the procedure. *Via falsa* may occur when probing is performed forcefully. The endoscopic view of the stent leaving the common canaliculus confirms its situation (Fig. 5.7). Placement of the stent does not change the final outcome, however, it facilitates post-operative care and impedes fibrous closure: with the endoscope one can "follow" the stent up towards the common canaliculus. Furthermore, it enables the drainage of the eye drops.

The mucosal flap is then repositioned (Fig. 5.8) with the intent to cover as much denuded bone as possible and paying attention to keep both proximal ends of the silicone probe towards the septum avoiding their positioning below the flap. The catheter is then fixed on the outer skin of the nose. In children knotting the probe inside the nose prevents from manipulations. Before doing so, it is important to check if both eyelids can be opened completely (Fig. 5.9).

Intranasal packing, using a reduced Merocel (usually a third of a normal nasal packing) to fix the mucosal flap, is kept in place for 1 week after surgery (Fig. 5.10). Also, the same piece of Merocel helps to adapt the septal mucosa in cases of prior "miniseptoplasty."

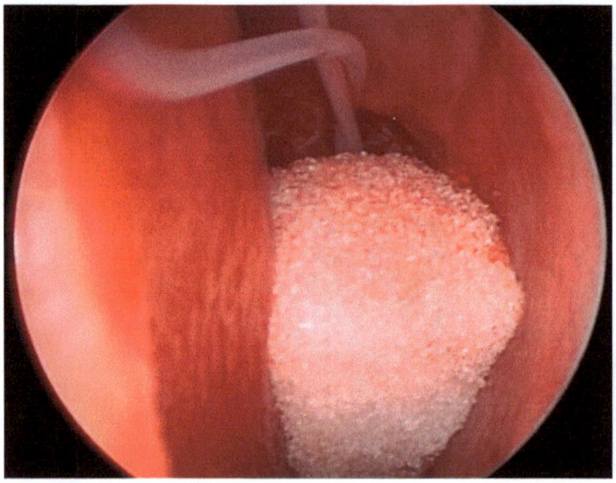

Fig. 5.10. Merocel helps to adapt the mucosal flap onto the lateral wall, also towards the septum in case of a miniseptoplasty

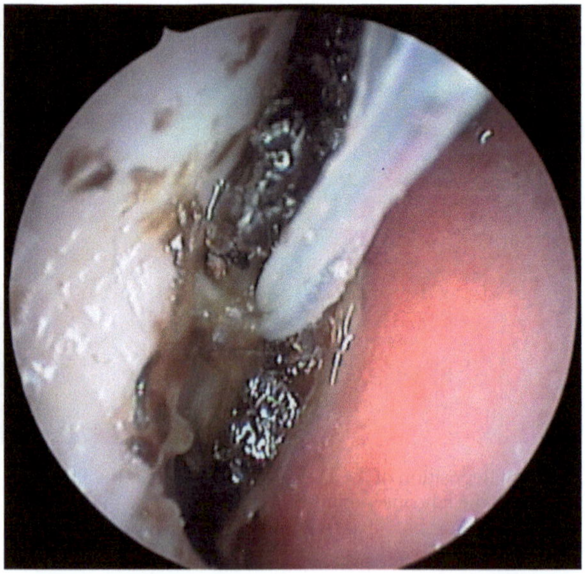

Fig. 5.11. Stenting allows to "follow" endoscopically the probe up to the opening of the sac, removing crusts and fibrin clots avoiding touching of the lateral aspect of the sac, which may produce pain

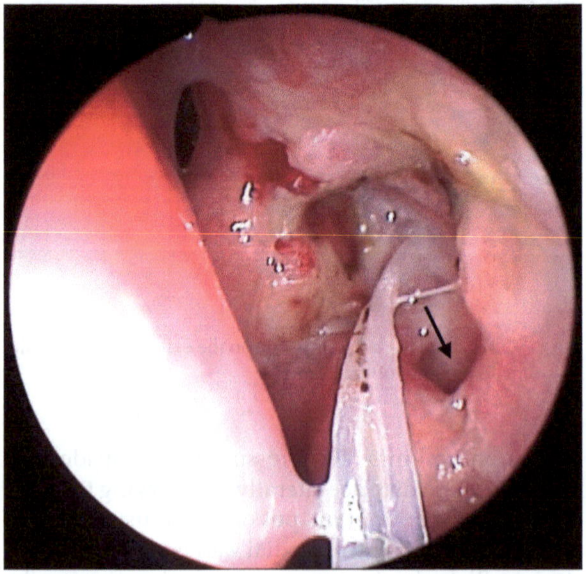

Fig. 5.12. Once the site has been cleaned, the opening of the sac may be observed. In this case, both ends of the silicone probe leave the common canaliculus and inferiorly the remnants of the sac remain open. Inflammation of the sac may lead to mucous formation and temporary obstruction of the common canaliculus (so-called lacrimal sump syndrome). A soft external massage may help to evacuate the mucous

5.5 Highlights

The important points are as follows:

1. Identification of the posterior edge of the maxillary crest before or after creating the inferiorly based mucosal flap
2. Sharp instruments to create the mucosal flap
3. Resection of the superior aspect of the maxillary crest to expose the common canaliculus
4. External fixation of the lacrimal sac from outside with the finger when making the incision
5. Careful probing of superior (more difficult) and inferior canaliculi to avoid "via falsa"
6. Control of sufficient opening of the eyelids before fixing the silicone probe

5.6 Immediate Post-operative Care and Follow-up

The piece of Merocel is removed between days 5 and 7 after surgery. This period seems to be enough to produce a steady scarring of the mucosal flap onto the partially exposed bony wound. Instead of just pulling the Merocel, it seems better to rotate it, to prevent laceration of the mucosal flap. On the left side, rotation should be performed counterclockwise, on the right side clockwise. Fibrin clots and crusts, if any, are

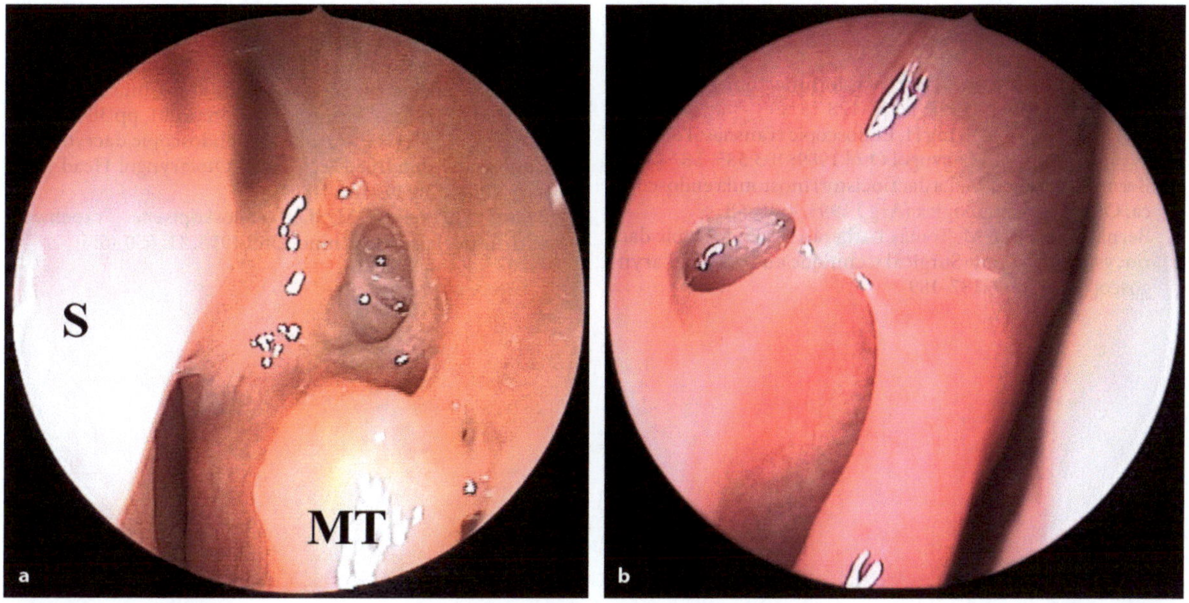

Fig. 5.13. a Left DCR after 12 weeks. Note minor granulations tissue at the superior edge, but patency of the DCR. Minor synechia of the head of the middle turbinate (*MT*) to the lateral wall. *S* septum. b Right patent DCR after more than 1 year

cleared every 7 days for the first 3 weeks after DCR (Figs. 5.11, 5.12). It is here where the silicone probe shows another advantage: with the endoscope one can follow it until the entrance of the lacrimal sac removing crusts and fibrin clots progressively and not touching the remnant lacrimal, which may be painful.

Patients are indicated to rinse their nose with saline once or twice a day from the second week onward. Patients are not allowed to blow their nose for 10 days after surgery and they are asked to perform regular gentle massages of the external aspect of the lacrimal sac (inner angle of the eye) to facilitate drainage. When sneezing, the mouth should be opened for about 10 days to prevent cheek or orbital emphysema. The silicone probes are removed after 2–3 weeks. Keeping the probes in place longer may produce granulation tissue formation at the surroundings of the common canaliculus. Our experience has shown that there is absolutely no need to keep silicone catheters for a longer period of time [7]. Eye drops containing steroids and antibiotics can be prescribed without any complications for 2–3 months at a low dosage of two drops every 8 h to provide continuous flow through the lacrimal system. After withdrawal of the probe, an endoscopy is performed 4–6 weeks later.

Intranasal application of topical steroids may be needed if other surgery has been performed in the nose or the paranasal sinuses, or when minor granulation tissue appears.

Sometimes, epiphora starts again during the follow-up. This may be secondary to collection of mucus in the remnant sac obstructing the drainage of the common canaliculus, which is known as "lacrimal sump syndrome" (Fig. 5.12). Soft external massage empties the sac. Once the scarring is completed, patients are visited 1 year later (Fig. 5.13).

Reference

1. Rice DH. Endoscopic dacryocystorhinostomy: a cadaver study. Am J Rhinol 1998; 2:127–128
2. McDonongh M, Meiring H. Endoscopic transnasal dacryocystorhinostomy. J Laryngol Otol 1989; 103:585–587
3. Bernal Sprekelsen M. La dacriocistorrinostomía endoscópica. Otorrinolaringológica (Arg.) 1995, 4:61–68
4. Bernal Sprekelsen M, Tomás Barberán M. Endoscopic dacriocystorhinostomy. Surgical technique and results. Laryngoscope 1996; 106:187–189
5. Bernal Sprekelsen, M. Resultados de la dacriocistorrinostomía endoscópica. In: Bernal Sprekelsen M, Massegur Solench H, Sprekelsen Gassó C, Ademá Alcover JM, Fabra JM, Moina H (eds) Cirugía endoscópica naso-sinusal. Básica y avanzada. Gráficas Alzamora, Gerona 2001, pp 304–308
6. Massegur H, Trias E, Adema JM. Endoscopic dacryocystorhinostomy: modified technique. Otolaryngol Head Neck Surg 2004; 130:39–46
7. Bernal Sprekelsen M. Die endoskopische Tränenwegschirurgie. Laryngo-Rhino-Otol 1998; 11: 650–651

Chapter 6

Dacryocystorhinostomy in Children

6

Manuel Bernal-Sprekelsen, Isam Alobid, Ferran Ballesteros,
Manuel Tomás-Barberán, David A. Della Rocca and R.C. Della Rocca

Core Messages

- There is a high tendency of about 85% of spontaneous relief of epiphora within the first 9 months of life.
- Malformations of the lacrimal pathways or other craniofacial malformations are more frequently associated than in adults.
- In unresolved congenital obstructions, dacryoceles, punctal agenesis, lacrimal fistula, post-traumatic, and post-inflammatory canalicular obstruction, no spontaneous opening can be expected.
- Indications of DCR in children below the age of 1 year are limited.
- Fixing a silicone catheter by putting several knots endonasally prevents manipulations.

Contents

6.1 Introduction

Many newborns suffer from congenital obstruction of the lacrimal pathways. The rate of congenital membranous stenosis of the lacrimal excretory systems in newborns has been reported to be as high as 50% [1]. Fortunately, there is a high rate of spontaneous relief of the epiphora within the first 9 months of life [2]; thus, repair of a lacrimal duct obstruction should rarely be done prior to this age. The majority of these congenital lacrimal duct obstructions can be managed well with nasolacrimal probing and intubation. These techniques are reviewed in Chap. 5.

6.2 Indications and Contraindications

Beyond the common causes of epiphora due to an abnormality of the distal lacrimal excretory system, abnormalities of the lacrimal canaliculus, common canaliculus, and lacrimal sac can often only be definitively repaired with a dacryocystorhinostomy (DCR). These abnormalities include dacryocystitis, chronic dacryocystocele, amniocystocele, punctal agenesis, lacrimal fistulization, and common canalicular scarring. Also, epiphora due to a congenital lacrimal duct obstruction that has not improved with appropriate probing techniques might necessitate a DCR.

Notably, lacrimal excretory system obstructions secondary to larger craniofacial abnormalities could indicate the need for more extensive evaluation and reconstruction of the bony and soft tissue anatomy [3, 4].

The results of dacryocystorhinostomies have been quite good for a variety of etiologies. A large study by Barnes et al. [3] has shown an excellent response of congenital lacrimal duct obstruction, refractory to lacrimal intubation, to the external DCR technique. Among 134 cases among 121 patients, 96% had a complete cure of their symptoms while all of the patients had improvement of their epiphora. Using similar techniques, another study showed a 90% cure with dacryocystitis as the etiology [5].

A study by Bernal-Sprekelsen et al. did show good results from endonasal DCR in a series of 24 children on 31 sides with a mean age of 5.6 years (2–14 years). After a primary endonasal DCR, there was a patency rate of 90.3%, which improved to 100% after a revision [6]. Indications for surgery included relapsing dacryocystitis (*n*=22), epiphora (*n*=7), and two dacryoceles. Twenty-eight of 31 sides remained patent at 1 year of follow-up [7].

With cases of abnormal bony anatomy, or longstanding dacryocystitis with extensive scarring, the transcutaneous approach to a DCR is indicated as it gives superior visualization of the lacrimal sac and medial orbital wall anatomy.

Other studies have shown poorer results when canalicular obstruction is seen [7]. The presence of such a malformation might necessitate a conjunctival dacryocystorhinostomy with a Jones tube [8]; however, the need for careful follow-up and the possibility of tube migration or extrusion should be stressed to the patient's family. We recommend this type of procedure only at or after 8 years of age. An alternative technique is a DCR with canaliculaplasty and silicone tube intubation, which better approximates the normal anatomy and eliminates the complication of late Jones tube migration. In cases of DCR with canalicular intubation only, the results were also good (79%).

6.3 Surgical Technique

Endoscopic DCR and external DCR in children are procedures that can be successful with a surgeon's deep knowledge of the anatomy of the orbital wall, soft tissue system, and nasal passage. The exposure and technique of the pediatric DCR is similar to that of an adult. Detailed descriptions of DCR techniques in the adult patient are described in previous chapters and are not repeated in this chapter.

In the pediatric age group the nasal passages are very narrow; therefore, endoscopic DCR in small children can be a technically difficult procedure. Surgery under a microscope may provide an enlarged working field if a self-retaining speculum is used. It is important to stress that if the endonasal anatomy is prohibitive, improved exposure of the lacrimal sac, lacrimal bone, and maxillary bones should be obtained through a transcutaneous incision at the anterior lacrimal crest.

Fixation of the tube to the nasal wall is poorly tolerated by young children and can cause constant irritation. A series of five single ties of the silicone tube left to freely lie within the nose is a good alternative. The tied knot should regress 12–15 mm deep into the nares.

6.4 Special Instrumentation

In children under 1 year of age, a 2.7-mm endoscope might be a better fit into the nose than a 4-mm scope. Also, handling a hammer and chisel might be difficult and dangerous in a narrow nose. Kerrison rongeurs (Karl Storz, Germany) with a 1-mm bite are more suitable [9].

6.5 Complications and Postoperative Care

A potentially dangerous complication to a pediatric DCR is excessive perioperative and postoperative epistaxis. The blood volume of children and especially babies is small as compared with an adult. For this reason, excessive blood loss is less well tolerated. For persistent nasal bleeding fastidious nasal packing may be necessary.

In children, endoscopic removal of fibrin clots and crusts necessitates general anesthesia; therefore, the indication for such a procedure should be restricted; as such cases with a "second look" do not show an improved outcome [7]. Other postoperative complications include infection and granuloma formation. Postoperative oral antibiotics, such as amoxicillin (7 days) and a broad-spectrum antibiotic/steroid combination drop, should be used postoperatively (10–14 days)

6.6 Tube Removal (Dacryocystorhinostomy)

The silicone tube when placed should be kept in position for 12 weeks. The tube may be removed sooner if there is stretching of the punctum. The tube can be removed in the office only in a very cooperative child. A brief masked general anesthesia may be needed in most younger children. If the tube is visualized with an endoscope, it should be retrieved through the nares after it is cut at the medial commissure. If the tube is not identified, it can be retrieved through the superior punctum. An antibiotic and steroid combination eye drop is advised three to four times daily for 7–10 days following the tube removal.

Reference

1. Pau H. Ophthalmologische Aspekte bei Tränenwegsstenosen. Otorhinolaryngol Nova 1991; 1:221–226
2. Petersen RA, Robb RM. The natural course of congenital obstruction of the nasolacrimal duct. J Pediatr Ophthal Strabismus 1978; 15:246–250
3. Barnes EA, Abou-Rayyah Y, Rose GE. Pediatric dacryocystorhinostomy for nasolacrimal duct obstruction. Ophthalmology 2001; 108:1562–1564
4. Struck HG, Weidlich R. Indications and prognosis of dacryocystorhinostomy in childhood. A clinical study 1970–2000. Ophthalmologe 2001; 98:560–563
5. Welham RA, Hughes SM. Lacrimal surgery in children. Am J Ophthalmol 1985; 99:27–34
6. Bernal Sprekelsen M, Massegur H, Tomas M. Endoscopic sinus surgery in children. Rev Laryngol Otol Rhinol 2003; 124:245–250
7. Kominek P, Cervenka S. Pediatric endonasal dacryocystorhinostomy: a report of 34 cases. Laryngoscope 2005; 115:1800–1803
8. Hakin KN, Sullivan TJ, Sharma A, Welham RA. Paediatric dacryocystorhinostomy. Aust N Z J Ophthalmol 1994; 22:231–235
9. Bernal Sprekelsen M, Tomás Barberán M. Endoscopic dacryocystorhinostomy. Surgical technique and results. Laryngoscope 1996; 106:187–189

Chapter 7

Laser-Assisted Dacryocystorhinostomy 7

S. Mirza and N. Jones

Core Messages

- Make certain of a diagnosis of distal nasolacrimal duct obstruction as a DCR does not help proximal obstruction and is less effective if there is a functional problem.
- Although rare, it is important to exclude pathology such as malignancy in the nasolacrimal sac or paranasal sinuses. Results are poorer in sarcoidosis and surgery should be avoided in active Wegener's granulomatosis.
- Laser DCR has many advantages over conventional methods when a patient is anticoagulated or has a coagulopathy.
- Laser DCR is more amenable to being performed under local anesthetic than other techniques, which is useful in those patients unfit for a general anesthetic.
- Laser DCR can be used to resolve cases of acute dacryocystitis.
- A relative indication for laser DCR is for revision surgery for a failed external DCR when there is often only a thin membrane blocking the rhinostomy.
- Suitable lasers include the KTP/532, Holmium:YAG, and diode laser.
- Laser DCR long-term patency rates are generally not as good as external DCR or endoscopic DCR using conventional instruments.

Contents

7.1 Introduction and Background of Technique

A DCR involves the creation of a surgical opening between the lacrimal sac and the nasal fossa just posterior to the anterior lacrimal crest. This new opening is proximal to the site of obstruction in the nasolacrimal duct, and re-establishes the flow of lacrimal fluid into the nose. There are two approaches: external and transnasal. The transnasal approach can be performed by direct vision, microscope, or more commonly by the endoscope, and can be undertaken with cold instrumentation (chisel, drill, and power drill) or the laser.

The transnasal DCR was first described by Caldwell in 1893 (Caldwell 1893) but did not gain widespread acceptance due to poor illumination of the nasal cavity and intraoperative bleeding.

In the 1980s there was a renewed interest in the transnasal approach prompted by the general evolution of endonasal procedures such as functional endoscopic sinus surgery (FESS), and the introduction of vastly superior and reliable instrumentation.

Since its introduction into surgical practice, laser technology has improved the operative management of a number of procedures. In an attempt to achieve precise bone removal with meticulous hemostasis, the laser DCR was developed and first described by Massaro et al. (1990). Since then, there have been a number of series reported using various types of laser for DCR with variable results, as shown in Tables 7.1 and 7.2.

7.1.1 Types of Laser

The type of laser appropriate for a DCR would allow delivery via flexible optic fibers, achieve effective bone ablation and provide good hemostasis with a relatively shallow depth of penetration; therefore, the potassium titanyl phosphate (KTP/532), diode, and holmium:yttrium aluminium garnet (Ho:YAG) are suitable. The carbon dioxide (CO2) laser is not ideal due to its poor hemostatic properties, poor bone ablation, and cumbersome delivery system. The Argon laser also has relatively poor bone ablation.

The Ho:YAG laser fibers have multiple use specification and this can potentially reduce the cost per procedure. The major disadvantage is the splattering of tissue with soiling of the lens, requiring frequent cleaning and more collateral damage when compared with the KTP laser.

The KTP/532 with its star-pulse mode is most suitable as it vaporizes the bone effortlessly and without splattering. The diode laser also has sufficient power to ablate bone. The major disadvantage of the KTP and the diode laser is that the optical fiber is marketed for single use and therefore the cost per procedure for these lasers is significantly higher.

The literature reports success rates for the various lasers of around 60–80% (Woog et al. 1993; Kong et al. 1994; Boush et al. 1994; Sadiq et al. 1997; Mirza et al. 2002) with one report of a 99% success rate (Camara et al. 2000)

7.1.2 Laser vs Non-laser Endonasal DCR

The endonasal laser DCR (ELDCR) is similar to the cold-instrument endonasal DCR (EDCR) technique with the exception that laser energy is used to vaporize the mucosa and ablate the bone to create a fistula; however, the success rates following non-laser EDCR are somewhat higher with a number of studies quoting success rates of over 90% (Weidenbecher et al. 1994; Sprekelsen and Barberan 1996; Yung and Hardman-Lea 1999). The better surgical outcome with conventional surgery is related to a wider bony opening and it obviates the thermal damage caused by the laser which produces more fibrosis and occlusion at the rhinostomy site. The advantages and disadvantages of the laser technique are given in Table 7.3.

7.1.3 Team Approach

Close cooperation with ophthalmalogical colleagues is essential to ensure a correct diagnosis. Although the ELDCR is mainly an ENT-oriented procedure with most of the surgery being intranasal, it is ideal if

Table 7.1. List of laser DCR series

Reference	Laser	Number	Success (%)	Comments
Massaro et al. (1990)	Argon	1	100	Microscope
Gonnering et al. (1992)	CO2, KTP	15	100	
Reifler (1993)	KTP	19	68	
Woog et al. (1993)	Ho:YAG	40	82	With drill
Metson et al. (1994)	Ho:YAG	34	85	
Seppa et al. (1994)	CO2/Nd:YAG	12	83	Microscope
Kong et al. (1994)	Ho:YAG, Nd:YAG	92	77–96% with revision	
Boush et al. (1994)	Argon	46	70–80% with revision	
Tutton and O'Donnell (1995)	Nd:YAG	6	100	Direct vision
Sadiq et al. (1996)	Ho:YAG	50	70	
Hehar et al. (1997)	Ho:YAG	50	70	
Sadiq et al. (1997)	Ho:YAG	97	81	
Mickelson et al. (1997)	KTP	12	100	
Hartikainen et al. (1998)	CO2-Nd:YAG combined	32	63	Microscope
Szubin et al. (1999)	Argon, Ho:YAG	28	96	
Camara et al. (2000)	Ho:YAG	123	99	
Doyle et al. (2000)	KTP	6	0	Pediatric cases
Ibrahim et al. (2001)	Not stated	53	58	
Velegrakis et al. (2002)	CO2	53	96	Microscope
Piaton et al. (2002)	Diode	363	92	
Tripathi et al. (2002)	Ho:YAG	46	89	
Moore et al. (2002)	Ho:YAG	33	71	
Mirza et al. (2002)	KTP	76	64	
Liu et al. (2003)	Nd:YAG	227	93–96	
Morgan et al. (2004)	Ho:YAG	9	67	
Bakri et al. (2003)	Ho:YAG	201	63–76	

All series were performed endoscopically unless otherwise stated

Table 7.2. Lasers used for endonasal laser DCR

KTP
Holmium:YAG
Diode
Neodymium:YAG
Argon
CO_2

Table 7.3. The advantages and disadvantages of the laser endonasal DCR over non-laser endonasal DCR

Advantages	Disadvantages
Can be performed under local anesthetic	Lower success rate
Can be performed on anticoagulated patients	Expensive equipment
Shorter operative time	Laser precautions required
More effective hemostasis and low hemorrhage rates	

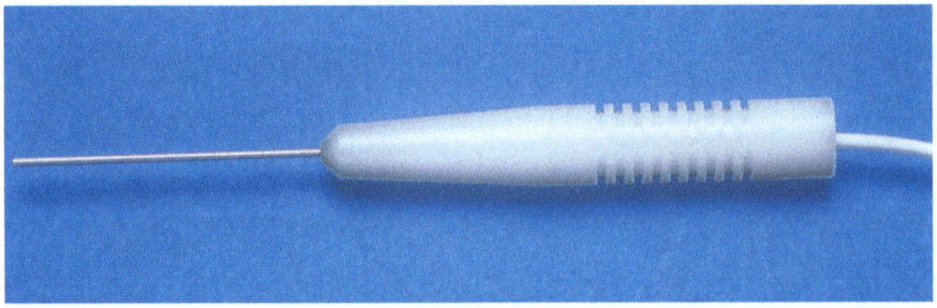

Fig. 7.1. Line diagram represents the method used in laser DCR

an otorhinolaryngologist and ophthalmologist undertake the procedure jointly. Assistance from the ophthalmologist to pass a vitreo-retinal light pipe to transilluminate the site of the operation is useful (Fig. 7.1), and some patients may have additional pathology such as a stenosed punctum, which requires concurrent management by way of a three-snip procedure.

7.2 Indications for Endoscopic Laser Dacryocystorhinostomy

Dacryocystorhinostomy (DCR) is indicated for significant symptoms such as epiphora due to nasolacrimal duct obstruction which is not relieved by simple probing and syringing. It is not indicated for sole obstruction in the puncti, canaliculi, common duct, and lacrimal sac. In many patients there is some proximal obstruction associated with distal blockage. In such cases, gentle probing and dilatation in conjunction with a DCR and insertion of stents can be performed, although the results of such an approach are not as favorable as cases of pure distal blockage. The laser DCR can also be used in cases of acute dacryocystitis complicated by abscess formation (Morgan et al. 2004). The laser DCR is ideal when a patient is anticoagulated or has a coagulopathy. Not only does it avoid any disruption to their anticoagulant therapy, but it can also be done as a day-case procedure (Smithard et al. 2003). It is also more amenable to being performed under local anesthetic than other techniques, which is useful in those patients unfit for a general anesthetic. A relative indication for laser DCR is revision surgery for a failed external DCR (Szubin et al. 1999). An external DCR may be unsuccessful for several reasons, but predominantly it is due to excessive scarring that is often only a thin membrane blocking the rhinostomy. Revision surgery can be performed effectively with the laser, removing the scarred tissue bloodlessly, although the outcome cannot be reliably predicted on account of excessive scarring which may involve the canaliculi and the common canaliculus. It is important that during the procedure the laser power setting be high enough to effect vaporization, rather than charring, since the latter will mean that further laser energy and heat may be dissipated to surrounding tissue and produce more scar tissue.

7.3 Contraindications for Endoscopic Laser Dacryocystorhinostomy

The endonasal approach is inappropriate in the presence of malignant lesions of the lacrimal system or the surrounding tissues. In active Wegener's granulomatosis any instrumentation induces marked adhesions and stenosis, and a DCR by any method is contraindicated. Dacryoliths usually require an external approach for removal. A relative contraindication is a history of trauma as the bone medial to the sac may be thick. The indications and contraindications for laser DCR are summarized in Table 7.4.

Table 7.4. Indications and contraindications for laser DCR

Indications for laser DCR
Distal nasolacrimal duct obstruction
Acute dacryocystitis
Revision surgery for failed external DCR
Patients unfit for a general anesthetic
Patients with a coagulopathy
Contraindications
Tumors of lacrimal system
Wegener's granulomatosis
Abnormally thick bone (e.g., nasoethmoid trauma)
Lacrimal sac pathology

7.4 Patient Assessment: Case History

Syringing and probing of the lacrimal system is used to diagnose the site of any nasolacrimal duct obstruction. Nasendoscopy prior to ELDCR is advisable to ensure adequate access and rule out co-existing pathology.

Patients with epiphora may have one or more sites of obstruction along the lacrimal drainage pathway. Proximal obstruction needs to be excluded before listing a patient for ELDCR and this can be performed without the need for complex investigations in the majority of cases. It is also important to exclude malignancy, which may present with blood stained epiphora, or a progressively enlarging mass within the lacrimal sac with or without tethering of the skin. A thorough ophthalmic and nasal examination usually fails to show any obvious etiological factor in the majority of cases.

A history of trauma to the nasoethmoid complex, such as a LeFort type-II or type-III fracture, may result in an unfavorable outcome from EDCR. Such cases are best dealt with via an external DCR where wide excision of bone and mucosa can be undertaken under direct vision.

A visible and palpable swelling, infero-lateral to the medial canthus, may indicate the presence of a lacrimal mucocele or pyocele. Massaging of the lacrimal sac may express discharge or frank pus from the puncti, indicating a diagnosis of mucoid or purulent dacryocystitis.

The patency of the system is tested by flushing with saline solution. Flushing should be undertaken gently since it can cause damage to the delicate canaliculi and produce false passages. Syringing and probing is done via the upper canaliculus with one of the following results:

1. No obstruction = functional problem. In the absence of obstruction, the saline passes down the system into the nose and the oropharynx where a salty taste is experienced. The epiphora may be due to a malposition, where the punctum is not in contact with the conjunctiva of the eyelid, or an inadequate lacrimal pump. Scintigraphy may help confirm the diagnosis.
2. An inability to enter the punctum or cannaliculus = proximal blockage. This can be due to a stenosed punctum, canaliculi, or both. Examination of the punctum may show it to be extremely small. If the lower canaliculus is stenosed, a DCR is of little value as 90% of tears drain via this route. Probing the lacrimal pathway with a smooth double-ended Bowman's probe often has a "soft stop" as the probe passes through the common canaliculus (Fig. 7.2). In some cases, probing and dilatation may be successful in re-establishing the patency of the system or with a stenosed punctum the ophthalmologist may do a "three-snip procedure" to enlarge the opening.
3. Regurgitation of fluid on syringing through the upper punctum = distal blockage

If saline regurgitates through the lower punctum after a slight delay, then it must have entered the lacrimal sac, encountered a distal obstruction, and returned through the upper canaliculus. The positive regurgitation test thus confirms an obstruction in the nasolacrimal duct. Rarely, a minor degree of blockage of the nasolacrimal duct may resolve with flushing.

Some cases present with both proximal as well as distal obstruction. When the proximal obstruction is

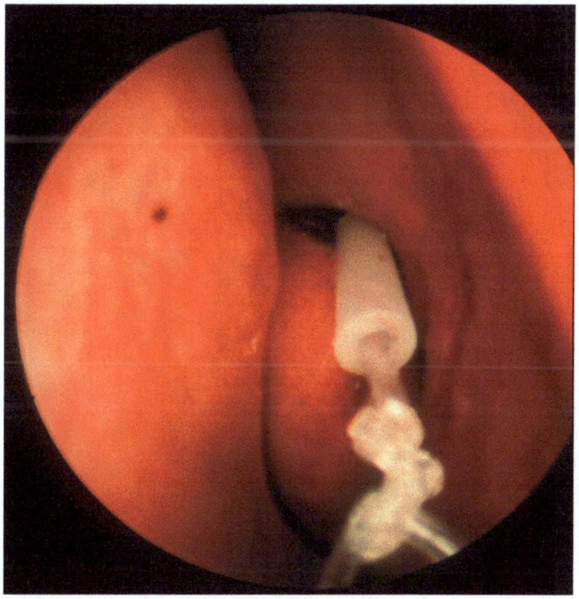

Fig. 7.2. Lacrimal probing of the inferior canaliculus just before passing it through the common canaliculus where a "soft stop" is felt

solely due to a stenosed punctum, a simultaneous three-snip procedure forms an integral part of the ELDCR. The endonasal DCR is inadvisable in concurrent significant proximal obstruction, since the results are invariably disappointing.

Endoscopic examination of the nasal passage is performed to ensure adequate access to the operation site by excluding, among others, a markedly deviated nasal septum, nasal polyposis, chronic rhinosinusitis, and neoplastic lesions. If any nasal conditions are found, then a preliminary or concurrent management of such conditions is planned with the proposed DCR. Surgery is contraindicated in active Wegener's granulomatosis.

7.4.1 Investigations

Computed tomography scanning is not routinely performed unless there is suspicion of neoplasm. A dacryocystogram has an associated risk of trauma, requires an experienced radiologist, and yields little additional information that could influence the patient's management and is therefore not routinely performed.

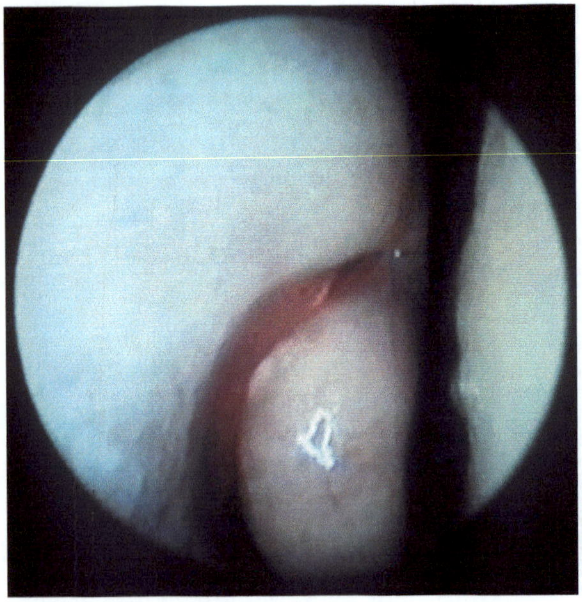

Fig. 7.3. A vitreoretinal light pipe

7.5 Instrumentation

The instruments used are as follows: endoscopes 0°, 4 mm (Storz) / microscope; Laser-Orion Laser System KTP/532 with 0.4-mm fiber; Robinson's laser handpiece (Laserscope); Vitreo retinal light pipe (Disposable endoilluminator, Infinitec, Chesterfield, Mo.; Fig. 7.3); canaliculi probes ; and FESS instruments (Storz).

7.6 Anesthesia

The operation can be performed under either local or general anesthesia as per patient and surgeon preference.

7.6.1 Local Anesthetic

Amethocaine 1% drops are instilled into the conjunctival fornices. Both lids are infiltrated with lignocaine 1% with 1:200,000 adrenaline. A short length of 1 cm nasal packing soaked in 10 ml of Moffatts solution, consisting of 2 ml of 6% cocaine, 1 ml of 1:1000 adrenaline, 1 ml 8.4% sodium bicarbonate, and 6 ml normal saline (in a 70-kg adult), is placed into the nasal cavity and removed after 5 min, or alternatively cophenylcaine [lignocaine hydrochloride 5% w/v (50 mg) and phenylephrine hydrochloride 0.5% (5 mg) is used].

7.6.2 General Anesthetic

Local anesthetic as detailed above is still used in order to reduce intraoperative bleeding.

7.6.3 Operative Technique

Our preferred technique using the KTP/532 laser on star-pulse mode with a power setting of 50 W, 10 ms, and 10/s for soft tissue; and 70 W, 5 ms, and 20 pulses per second for bone.

7.6.3.1 Preparation

The patient is placed in the supine position at 15° reverse Trendelenburg. Appropriate laser-safety precautions for the patient and operating team are taken to avoid ocular injury. Wet eyepads are placed over the patient's eyes.

7.6.3.2 Access to the Operating Site

The nasal operating site is accessed either with the microscope or the endoscope. When the operating microscope is used, the 300-mm objective is further away from the operating site and thus remains soil-free. It also provides useful magnification. A Killian's speculum is placed in the nostril and the transilluminated site is located. The use of the microscope is, however, cumbersome and can add significantly to the operating time in inexperienced hands. Endoscopy with video monitoring is much more popular due to its superior visualization and it is easier to manipulate, though the lens gets soiled due to smoke, blood and debris. Frequent cleaning is required, particularly when using the Holmium:YAG laser. The 0° endoscope is adequate in most cases although the 45° endoscope may afford a better view into the sac. Each approach has its advantages and the choice would depend on individual training, preferences and the availability of equipment and dedicated instruments.

7.6.3.3 Insertion of the Light Pipe

The upper punctum is dilated and the vitreo retinal light pipe inserted. The pipe is advanced, initially in a vertical direction through the punctum for a millimeter or so, and then horizontally along the canaliculus towards the medial canthus. Some resistance is then felt at the common canaliculus (the soft stop) before it touches the mucosa of the medial wall of the sac (hard stop). From the hard stop, the pipe is withdrawn slightly and advanced in an inferior–medial slanting direction so that it passes into the lacrimal sac. The light is inserted into the upper punctum as it is easier to position the light pipe in the inferior part of the lacrimal sac. This helps placement of the rhinostomy in a dependent position obviating the formation of lacrimal sump syndrome (a blind pouch with collection of mucus and recurrent dacryocystitis). Canulating the upper canaliculus also obviates injuring the functionally more important inferior canaliculus. The light is then held in the most dependent position where its position can be seen intranasally. It must be kept in the same position while the rhinostomy is being made to avoid firing the laser in several positions when the light has moved.

7.6.3.4 Localization of the Transilluminated Site

If the light pipe is accurately positioned in the lacrimal sac, it is usually seen as a bright and sharp spot illumination underneath the tissues, just anterior to the attachment of the bony middle turbinate to the lateral nasal wall (Fig. 7.4). The area of maximal brightness corresponds with the posterior end of the lacrimal sac where the overlying bone is thinnest, not the center of the sac. Another landmark for sac location is the maxillary line, a bony eminence which extends from the anterior attachment of the middle turbinate to the root of the inferior turbinate. It overlies the maxillary–lacrimal suture line within the lacrimal fossa. The light of the endoscope may need to be reduced to accurately visualize the spot if there is an agger nasi cell which occurs in this position in approximately 8% of patients (Fig. 7.5). The mucosa of the transilluminated area is infiltrated with 0.25 ml of 1% lignocaine with 1:200,000 adrenaline using a dental syringe and needle.

7.6.3.5 Laser Vaporization of Mucosa and Bone

The laser optical fiber is taken to the operation site through a handpiece. Some handpieces contain a second channel that is used to evacuate smoke and debris generated at the operation site. The distal end of the handpiece may be bent by about 25° so that the beam is directed laterally. For the KTP and Ho:YAG lasers the laser probe is maintained in near contact mode during the procedure and the endoscope tip is positioned approximately 2–3 cm from the target site. The transilluminated area of mucosa covering the medial lacrimal bone is vaporized and then continued through the bone to make a shallow pit about 4–5 mm in diameter. The transillumination becomes brighter as the bone is thinned. The difficulty of this step de-

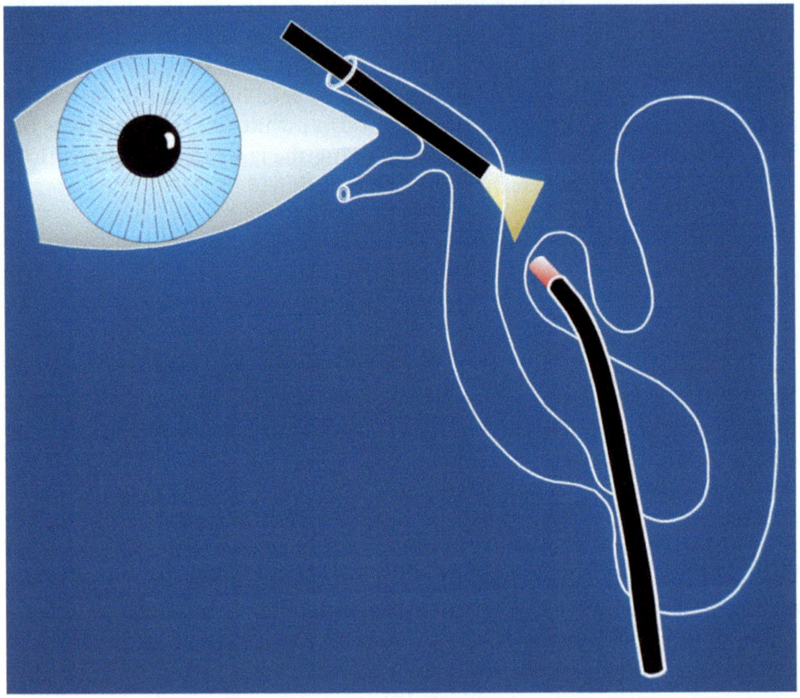

Fig. 7.4. Endoscopic view of the transilluminated lateral nasal wall indicates the site of the lacrimal sac

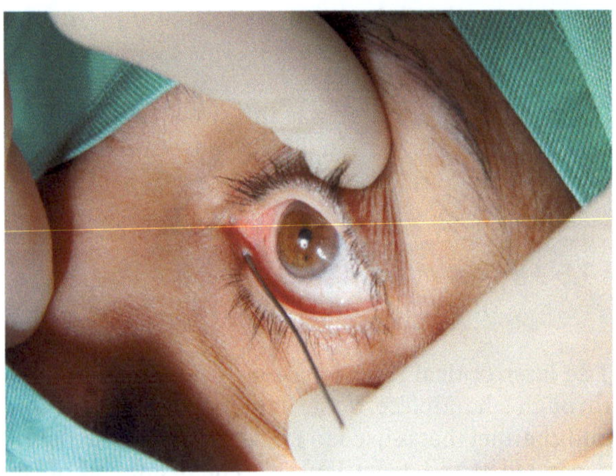

Fig. 7.5. Endonasal view shows diffuse light from within the lacrimal sac due to the presence of an agger nasi cell

pends on the thickness of the bone formed by the nasofrontal process of the maxilla. Posterior to the anterior lacrimal crest resection of the paper-thin lacrimal bone is easier. Bleeding can usually be arrested by using the laser in defocused mode. The vaporization is continued until an opening of around 5–8 mm in diameter is created in the center of the thinned-out bone. The laser cannot ablate charred tissue and so with continued use on such tissue heat is dissipated through the surrounding tissues increasing thermal injury.

7.6.3.6 Opening of the Lacrimal Sac and Creation of the Rhinostomy

The next step is to make an opening into the lacrimal sac. Movement of the light probe will confirm the location of the sac wall. The mucosa of the lacrimal sac is vaporized, again in the direction of transillumination. Alternatively, at this stage, a probe is passed into the lacrimal sac and the mucosa tented medially, into the bony opening to confirm the location of the sac. On breaching the lacrimal sac mucosa a fistula (rhinostomy) is created between the nasal cavity and the lacrimal sac. Various measuring devices can be used to assess the size of the rhinostomy to ensure uniformity. The rhinostomy should be at least 5 mm and preferably 10 mm in diameter to reduce the possibility of subsequent closure. Furthermore, the rhinostomy should be located as low as possible as a high rhinostomy results in a sump syndrome, predisposing to recurrent infections of the sac and the duct. A Dundas Grant attic seeker can be used to palpate the sac through the rhinostomy opening to ensure that there is no pocketing of mucus or pus, or fibrous strands, within the sac.

7.6.3.7 Syringing the System

The light pipe is removed and the lacrimal system flushed to ensure its free flow into the nasal cavity via the fistula. Forcible syringing should be avoided. Unsuccessful syringing indicates an additional proximal obstruction that may have been overlooked at the initial assessment.

7.6.3.8 Insertion of the Stent

A silicone tubed stent is used by a number of surgeons to maintain the patency of the rhinostomy (Woog et al. 1993; Reifler 1993; Szubin et al. 1999; Mirza et al. 2002). One end of the tubing is inserted and fed through the upper canaliculus, and the other through the lower canaliculus, so that the ends come out of the new opening into the nasal cavity. The ends are held in situ by a Watzke sleeve or they are gently tied so that a small loop remains at the inner canthus (Fig. 7.6). It is best to avoid excessive tightening of the loop as this may eventually cause "cheese wiring" at the medial canthus. Stents are removed by cutting the loop at the inner canthus and pulling the sleeve with stents from the nostril.

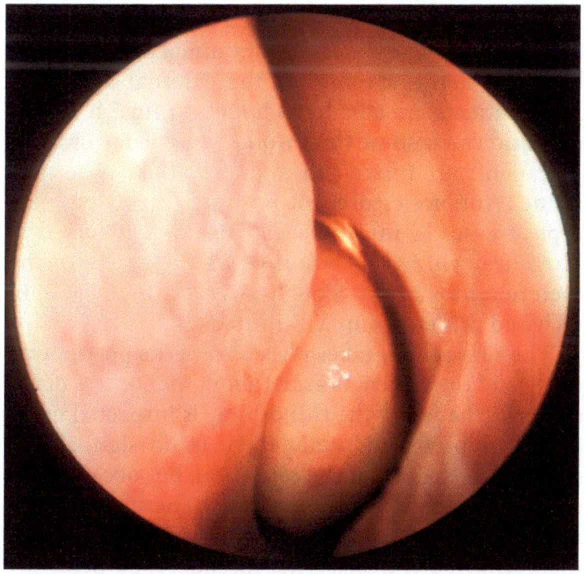

Fig. 7.6. Endonasal view shows the nasolacrimal stent and Watzke sleeve in position

7.7 Potential Problems

7.7.1 Narrow Punctum

Narrow punctum may require repeated careful dilatation before the light pipe can be passed. Significant trauma to the punctum and the canaliculus will lead to scarring, obstruction, and failure with persisting epiphora.

7.7.2 Poor Surgical Access

To obtain adequate access for the operation anatomical obstruction, such as a deviated nasal septum, prominent anterior lacrimal crest, or a large anterior end of the middle turbinate, may need initial surgical intervention.

7.7.3 Intraoperative Bleeding

One major advantage of the laser is its ability to secure intraoperative hemostasis. Bleeding can occur intraoperatively, but it is rarely troublesome. Minor bleeding can be controlled with a few laser strikes in defocused mode. Any bleeding which is not easily controlled by a few laser strikes in a defocused mode should be controlled with application of topical decongestants or vasoconstrictors on pledgets.

7.7.4 Aiming Beam Reflection

The reflection of the laser aiming beam from the tissues can be strong and this has the potential to be mistaken for the transilluminated light pipe beam with consequent vaporization undertaken at the incorrect site. It is often helpful to intermittently point the aiming beam away from the operating site and check the position of the light pipe in the sac.

7.7.5 Poor Transilluminated Light Beam Spot

The transillumination spot is not always easy to locate. Its location may be aided by further manipulation of the light pipe. Even if the light is located, it may be diffuse rather than bright and sharply demarcated, due to a number of factors:

1. Hypertrophied anterior end of middle turbinate. Enlargement of the soft tissue covering the anterior end of the middle turbinate may obscure part of the beam and need to be gently medialized. The middle turbinate is very sensitive, and if the procedure is done under local anesthetic, the middle turbinate will need anesthetizing before it is medialized.
2. Thick mucosa. The mucosa covering the anterior lacrimal crest may be thick and require vaporization before the transilluminated light becomes brighter. The mucosa of the lacrimal sac may be very thick as in cases of dacryolithiasis or a dacryomucocele. Laser vaporization should proceed with caution in order to avoid damaging the lateral wall of the sac.
3. Agger nasi anterior ethmoid cells. In approximately 8% of cases, there are agger nasi anterior ethmoid cells, between the sac and the nasal fossa. Uncapping the cell with the laser allows access to the bone that lies medial to the lacrimal sac.
4. Thick bone. In some young adults the bone can be thick and require extensive ablation to remove it. This is often a problem after trauma to the nasoethmoid complex and it is a relative indication for an external procedure. In these patients it is important to avoid charred bone accumulating as the laser will not be able to ablate it and its energy will be dissipated to the surrounding tissue and cause damage.

7.8 Highlights

The following points are important:

1. Dilate canaliculi. This should be performed gently to avoid iatrogenic injury.
2. Transilluminate the lacrimal sac. This should be performed gently and the light positioned at the inferior aspect of the lacrimal sac.
3. Creation of a rhinostomy: laser ablation of mucosa, bone, and the medial wall of the lacrimal sac. Regularly clean the operative field to avoid charring and thermal injury which predisposes to excessive scarring and closure of the rhinostomy resulting in failure. A rhinostomy of at least 5 mm (preferably 10 mm) should be formed.
4. Syringing. This confirms the patency of the system.
5. Stenting. To maintain rhinostomy patency until it is epithelialized.

7.9 Post-operative Care

Laser DCRs are usually performed as an outpatient procedure under local anesthesia. Post-operatively the rhinostomy site does not require regular surgical debridement. Patients are usually remarkably well following a laser DCR performed under either a local or general anesthesia. There is minimal discomfort or bruising of the eye, unlike the external approach. Most patients are able to go home within 2 h of surgery and can resume their work within a day or two.

Patients are instructed to douche their nose with saline. Antibiotics are not routinely prescribed, except in cases of infection. Patients are instructed to avoid heavy lifting, bending, or straining, or blowing their noses for 2 days. Slough covers the fistula within 48 h and this clears up within 10 days.

The first review takes place at 6 weeks post-operatively and the patient is asked about the success of the surgery. The site of the rhinostomy is inspected using a nasoendoscope. Usually there is no sign of any crusting at the site of the operation, but occasionally some granulation tissue is present. The stents are removed by cutting the loop between the canaliculi and then removed transnasally. An endoscope helps the stent to be located, although the patient may blow it out themselves.

After 3 months, the fistula cannot always be detected as a distinct opening, and the operation site may show a slight dimple, or may even appear completely normal.

7.10 Results

Most failures occur in the first 18 months due to stenosis at the rhinostomy site, although late stenosis can occur up to 3 years after surgery. Subjective scoring by the patient is usually used to measure the outcome. In unilateral cases, it is common for the patient to compare the results of the operation with the "good" eye. In bilateral cases, the patient compares improvement with the severity of watering prior to the operation. In the immediate post-operative period, particularly when a stent is not inserted, the improvement is both immediate and dramatic. As the healing proceeds, the symptoms may return, but less so in both severity and frequency. Where the improvement is partial, it is usual for the patient to complain of eye watering in cold winds, or in the smoky atmosphere of bars and restaurants. In cases with no improvement whatsoever, however short-lived, there may be other reasons for failure such as atony of the lacrimal pump.

Endoscopic examination may show no patent rhinostomy, but in a number of cases, the patient remains symptom-free. It is likely that a minute opening, not easily visible to the naked eye, may remain patent and continue to drain. An alternative explanation for the improvement of symptoms when no patent stoma is seen, is that the pathology responsible for the distal obstruction has resolved.

A physiological and objective method to assess the patency of the stoma consists of the dye disappearing test where, for example, fluorescein is placed into the conjunctiva without any syringing of the puncti and canaliculi. A nasal endoscope then confirms the passage of the fluorescein into the nasal fossa signifying a patent system.

7.11 Management of Failures of Laser DCR

In cases which fail to improve after laser DCR, an accurate reassessment is conducted. The nose is examined for stenosis of the rhinostomy site or the presence of any synechia. Syringing and probing can help to define the patency of the system. The most common cause of failure is stenoses of the rhinostomy. In common with surgically created stomas in other parts of the body, the dacryocystorhinostomy also shrinks. The purpose of creating a large rhinostomy is to allow for the shrinkage but even so the nasal mucosa may grow over the bony opening and heal completely without any visible scarring. Other causes of obstruction of the internal nasal opening include granulations, adhesions, and synechia. Revision laser DCR surgery may be indicated and is easily performed with good success rates (Kong et al. 1994; Mirza et al. 2002). Some patients may ultimately require an external DCR.

7.12 Post-operative Complications

In the majority of patients, there are very few post-operative complications, and the procedure is associated with very low morbidity. A list of complications is given in Table 7.5 and the following is a brief summary of the more common ones.

Table 7.5. Complications of laser DCR

Stenosis
Granulation tissue
Synechia
Stent migration
Sump syndrome
Cutaneous fistula (rare)
Hemorrhage (rare)

7.12.1 Hemorrhage

Significant hemorrhage is rare in laser DCR, and only occasionally is nasal packing necessary, whereas with the external DCR it has been reported as occurring in 5–10% of patients.

7.12.2 Granuloma Formation

Rarely, granulations form at the site of the fistula. The most likely cause of granulation formation is a low-grade infection or a foreign body reaction to the stent if it rubs the rhinostomy site. Stent removal usually results in a satisfactory resolution. Antibiotic nasal and eye drops may help reduce the incidence of granulations.

7.12.3 Synechia

Synechia are adhesions that form between two damaged apposing mucosal surfaces and are not uncommon after nasal surgery. The damage may result from instrumentation or from the spread of laser thermal energy to surrounding non-target structures. Synechia usually form between the lateral surface of the middle turbinate and the medial surface of the lateral wall of the nose and may obstruct the rhinostomy resulting in failure of the procedure. Synechia occur more commonly in cases with narrow nasal fossa, large concha bullosas, and chronic pathological conditions of the nasal mucosa. If the synechae are symptomatic, then revision surgery may be required.

Covering the lateral surface of the middle turbinate with wet ribbon gauze during the procedure may prevent adhesions.

7.12.4 Stent Migration

An excessively tight stent may cut through the canaliculus as well as the skin in between them. The raw surfaces may heal with a web, which buries the stent. This usually results in scarring and may disrupt the lacrimal drainage pump system. A migrated stent can be retrieved from the nose by cutting one of the tubes that forms the loop before the sleeve or knot. Premature loss of silicone stents may also occur from the knot becoming loose.

7.13 Variations in the Standard Procedure

The success rate following the standard endonasal laser procedure described above is reported to be between 60 and 80%, depending upon the criteria used by various workers. In an effort to improve the success rate, various modifications have been introduced, some of which are briefly mentioned here.

7.13.1 Avoidance of Stenting

Most series have utilized stenting, and premature stent removal may be associated with failure (Boush et al. 1994; Sadiq 1997; Mirza et al. 2002); however, stenting may lead to complications such as the formation of granuloma, infection, or scarring of the lacrimal puncta, and therefore some authors advise avoiding routine stenting (Allen and Berlin 1989). Stenting may be particularly useful where there is considerable scarring from previous operations, and in revision endonasal surgery. The stent should be secured with a loose knot or a Watzke sleeve rather than metal clip in order to avoid a foreign body reaction and subsequent granuloma formation leading to fibrosis.

7.13.2 Combined Laser and "Cold" Instrument Surgery

Concomitant use of instruments such as the otodrill and microrongeur may be more effective in removing thick bone and less painful for the patient (Kong et al. 1994). In addition, using endoscopic instruments instead of laser vaporization to open the lacrimal sac may reduce scarring and improve patency rates (Szubin et al. 1999).

7.13.3 Antimitotic Application

Some surgeons advocate mitomycin C, an antimitotic agent, used as a topical application to discourage cell proliferation so as to reduce the amount of mucosal scar tissue that is the commonest cause of failure (Camara et al. 2000). You and Fang (2001) found that the topical application of mitomycin C was beneficial in patients undergoing an external DCR yet Zilelioglu et al. (1998) found it to be of no benefit. The only study of an antimetabolite in laser DCR was by Bakri et al. (2003) who found that the topical application of 5 FU failed to increase the patency rates in ELDCR.

7.14 Conclusion

The primary indication for the use of lasers in dacryocystorhinostomy is in patients with a coagulopathy, as the procedure can be done without the need for stopping any anticoagulant or any hematological intervention. Laser endonasal DCR can readily be done under local anesthetic as an outpatient procedure, but the incidence of restenosis is approximately 10% more than if conventional instruments are used. In revision DCR, a laser DCR can be done very easily as it usually only requires ablation of scar tissue that has formed at the rhinostomy site.

Reference

Allen KM, Berlin AJ. Dacryocystorhinostomy failure: association with nasolacrimal silicone intubation. Ophthalmic Surg 1989;20:486–489

Bakri K, Jones NS, Downes R, Sadiq SA. Intraoperative fluorouracil in endonasal laser dacryocystorhinostomy. Arch Otolaryngol Head Neck Surg 2003;129:233–235

Boush GA, Lemke BN, Dortzbach RK. Results of endonasal laser-assisted dacryocystorhinostomy. Ophthalmology 1994;101:955–959

Caldwell GW. Two new operations for obstruction of the nasal duct with preservation of the canaliculi and an incidental description of a new lacrimal probe. New York Med J 1893;573–581

Camara JG, Bengzon AU, Henson RD. The safety and efficacy of mitomycin C in endonasal endoscopic laser-assisted dacryocystorhinostomy. Ophthal Plast Reconstr Surg. 2000;16:114–118

Doyle A, Russell J, O'Keefe M. Paediatric laser DCR. Acta Ophthalmol Scand 2000;78:204–205

Gonnering RS, Lyon DB, Fisher JC. Endoscopic laser-assisted lacrimal surgery. Am J Ophthalmol 1991;111:152–157

Hartikainen J, Grenman R, Puukka P, Seppa H. Prospective randomized comparison of external dacryocystorhinostomy and endonasal laser dacryocystorhinostomy. Ophthalmology 1998;105:1106–1113

Hehar SS, Jones NS, Sadiq SA, Downes RN. Endoscopic holmium:YAG laser dacryocystorhinostomy: safe and effective as a day-case procedure. J Laryngol Otol 1997;111:1056–1059

Ibrahim HA, Batterbury M, Banhegyi G, McGalliard J. Endonasal laser dacryocysto-rhinostomy and external dacryocystorhinostomy outcome profile in a general ophthalmic service unit: a comparative retrospective study. Ophthalmic Surg Lasers 2001;32:220–227

Kong YT, Kim TI, Kong BW. A report of 131 cases of endoscopic laser lacrimal surgery. Ophthalmology 1994 101:1793–1800

Liu Y, Xiao J, Wang Y. Semiconductor laser use in endoscopic transnasal dacryocystorhinostomy. Lin Chuang Er Bi Yan Hou Ke Za Zhi 2002;16:594–595

Massaro BM, Gonnering RS, Harris GJ. Endonasal laser dacryocystorhinostomy: a new approach to nasolacrimal duct obstruction. Arch Ophthalmol 1990;108:1172–1176

Metson R, Woog JJ, Pulafito CA. Endoscopic laser dacryocystorhinostomy. Laryngoscope 1994;104:269–274

Mickelson SA, Kim DK, Stein IM. Endoscopic laser-assisted dacryocystorhinostomy. Am J Otolaryngol 1997; 18:107–111

Mirza S, Al-Barmani A, Douglas SA, Bearn MA, Robson AK. A retrospective comparison of endonasal KTP laser dacryocystorhinostomy versus external dacryocystorhinostomy. Clin Otolaryngol 2002;27:347–351

Moore WM, Bentley CR, Olver JM. Functional and anatomic results after two types of endoscopic endonasal dacryocystorhinostomy: surgical and holmium laser. Ophthalmology 2002;109:1575–1582

Morgan S, Austin M, Whittet H. The treatment of acute dacryocystitis using laser assisted endonasal dacryocystorhinostomy. Br J Ophthalmol 2004;88:139–141

Piaton JM, Keller P, Limon S, Quenot S. First line endonasal dacryocystorhinostomy technique and results. Comparison between diode laser and electrocautery instrument. Study based on 422 procedures. J Fr Ophtalmol 2002;25:135–145

Reifler DM. Results of endoscopic KTP laser-assisted dacryocystorhinostomy. Ophthal Plast Reconstr Surg 1993; 9:231–236

Sadiq SA, Hugkulstone CE, Jones NS, Downes RN. Endoscopic holmium:YAG laser dacryocystorhinostomy. Eye 1996;10:43–46

Sadiq SA, Ohrlich S, Jones NS, Downes RN. Endonasal laser dacryocystorhinostomy: medium-term results. Br J Ophthalmol 1997;81:1089–1092

Seppa H, Grenman R, Hartikainen J. Endonasal CO2-Nd:YAG laser dacryocysto-rhinostomy. Acta Ophthalmol (Copenh) 1994;72:703–706

Smithard A, Wynne D, Bingham BJ, Jones NS. Endonasal laser dacryocysto-rhinostomy: its role in anticoagulated patients. Laryngoscope 2003;113:1034–1036

Sprekelsen MB, Barberan MT. Endoscopic dacryocystorhinostomy: surgical technique and results. Laryngoscope 1996;106:187–189

Szubin L, Papageorge A, Sacks E. Endonasal laser-assisted dacryocysto-rhinostomy. Am J Rhinol 1999;13:371–374

Tripathi A, Lesser TH, O'Donnell NP, White S. Local anaesthetic endonasal endoscopic laser dacryocystorhinostomy: analysis of patients' acceptability and various factors affecting the success of this procedure. Eye 2002;16:146–149

Tutton MK, O'Donnell NP. Endonasal laser dacryocystorhinostomy under direct vision. Eye 1995;9:485–487

Velegrakis GA, Prokopakis EP, Panayotaki I, Pagalos AG, Siganos CS, Helidonis ES. Intranasal laser-assisted dacryocystorhinostomy with the use of a surgical microscope. Am J Otolaryngol 2002;23:272–276

Weidenbecher M, Hoseman W, Buhr W. Endoscopic endonasal dacryocystorhinostomy: results in 56 patients. Ann Otol Rhinol Laryngol 1994;103:363–367

Woog JJ, Metson R, Puliafito CA. Holmium:YAG endonasal laser dacryocysto-rhinostomy. Am J Ophthalmol 1993;116:1–10

You MW, Fang CT. Intraoperative mitomycin C in dacryocystorhinostomy. Ophthalmic Plast Reconstr Surg 2001; 17:115–119

Yung MW, Hardman-Lea S. Endoscopic inferior dacryocystorhinostomy. Clin Otol 1999;23:152–157

Zilelioglu G, Ugurbas SH, Anadolu Y, Akiner M, Akturk T. Adjunctive use of mitomycin C on endoscopic lacrimal surgery. Br J Ophthalmol 1998; 82:63–66

Chapter 8

Complications of Endoscopic DCR

8

Manuel Bernal-Sprekelsen, Isam Alobid and Joaquin Mullol Miret

Core Messages

- Minor complications of surgery of the lacrimal sac include mainly ecchymosis or emphysema of the cheek, burning of the skin of the nostril, and circumscribed exposure of the orbital fat.
- Major complications include bleeding into the orbit, lesion of the medial rectus muscle, and lacerations of the inferior canaliculus.
- Patients are carefully instructed not to blow their nose or to sneeze with their mouth open for a safety period of about 10 days after surgery. No tension should be applied to the silicone stent when it is fixed on the nose. Minor synechiae can be avoided preserving mucosa of the middle turbinate.

Contents

8.1 Introduction

Endonasal surgery of the lacrimal sac is performed in the anterior aspect of the nasal fossa. Therefore, the complication rate to be expected remains low; However, minor and major complications may occur. In this chapter, we present the most frequent complications, as well as how to prevent and treat them.

8.2 Classification of Complications of DCR

8.2.1 Minor Complications

Minor complications include mainly ecchymosis or emphysema of the cheek, both secondary to the resection of the limits of the lateral wall. Cheek ecchymosis may also occur if the soft tissues of the cheek are exposed, when the approach was too far anterior. In these cases bleeding may occur during the surgical procedure.

Also, dissection of the anterior aspect of the lacrimal sac may produce some bleeding intraoperatively due to the lesion of its anterior vessels; however, postoperative bleeding is rare and little if the surgery is limited to the lacrimal sac.

Burning of the skin may happen when the drill is in contact with the nostril during drilling. When the lacrimal sac is located more posteriorly, there might be a direct contact with the periorbit, even without the presence of a bony lamella between both; thus, when performing the incision of the lacrimal sac, the periorbit could be opened as well. Circumscribed exposure of the orbital fat usually has no consequences, if patients do not sneeze or blow their noses to prevent emphysema.

8.2.2 Major Complications

Bleeding into the orbit may occur. If the fixation of silicone stent on the nose has too much tension, lacerations of the inferior canaliculus may occur. Although this has no influence on the functional outcome, from the esthetic point of view it may be considered a major failure. Lesion of the medial rectus muscle of the orbit may lead to diplopia. Lesion of the anterior ethmoid artery is a complication of the additional ethmoid surgery; hence, also the bleeding into the orbit and its consequences.

8.3 Results

During our first experiences with endoscopic DCR our rate of minor complications was high, although without severe sequelae. In 1996 we published an incidence of ecchymosis of the cheek in 44%, subcutaneous emphysema in 9% and orbital emphysema in 2.6% [1]. Presently, these figures have been considerably reduced. We rarely see emphysemas at all, and if so, it is because the patient has sneezed with the mouth closed, or blown the nose before 1 week after surgery. Ecchymosis of the cheek appears from time to time especially in patients where the soft tissue of the cheek has been exposed before reaching the lacrimal sac. The rate of complications may be higher if extended surgery has been simultaneously performed; thus, Fayet et al. [2] report on moderate and severe intraoperative bleeding in 82 (27.3%) and 35 cases (11.6%), respectively, when an uncinectomy was included.

The hammer and chisel technique to remove the bone reports rate of minor intraoperative bleeding of about 18% (8 of 44 patients) [3].

Probably the most common minor complication reported has been postoperative eyelid hematoma in cases where orbital fat was exposed, which has happened in 12.5% of cases [4]. In our hands, inadvertent incision of the periorbita achieved a rate of 10.5% (16 patients) [1].

Dolman found 11 (5.5%) cases of epistaxis requiring perioperative nasal packing and inadvertent lesion of the periorbit in five patients. One patient reported transient diplopia after the medial rectus was inadvertently pulled [5]. In our series we had no such case.

Lesion of the sphincter of the canaliculi was not reported, although probing has been used in most

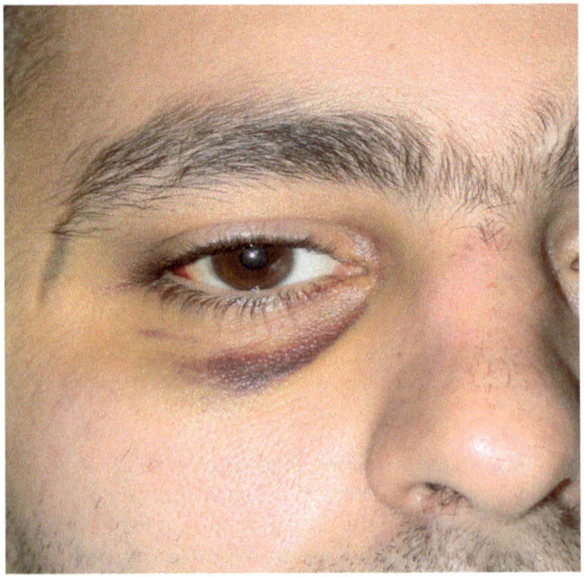

Fig. 8.1. Emphysema after DCR. Note the air in the inferior eyelid and in the conjunctiva. Spontaneous resolution may be expected. In cases with lacrimal sac infection prophylactic antibiotics should be prescribed. Courtesy Dr. Manuel Tomás, Mallorca, Spain

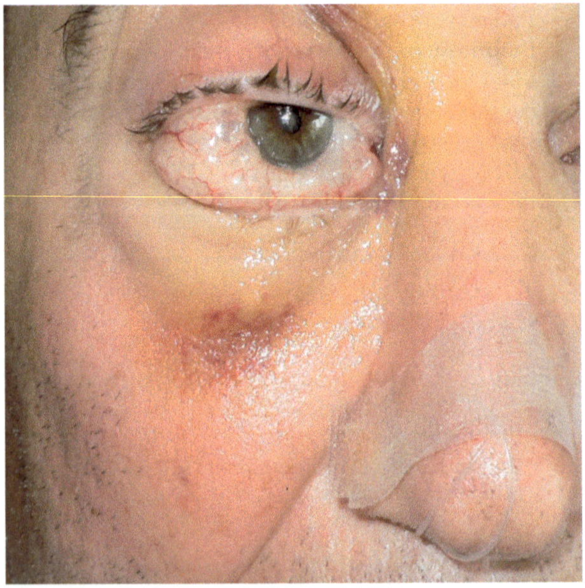

Fig. 8.2. Ecchymosis of the cheek after endoscopic DCR. Heparin ointment applied to the skin speed up the resorption

cases. A spontaneous retraction of the dilated sphincter can probably be assumed. Postoperative complications, such as eyelid ecchymosis, punctal granuloma, cyst of the punctum, or adhesion between the superior and inferior punctum, seem to be very rare [6]. Premature loss of silicone tube has no influence on the outcome.

Granulation tissue at the internal ostium can vary from 17.5 to 6.6% [1, 6]. Minor sinechiae between the head of the middle turbinate and the lateral wall has been observed in 22.4% of cases, with obliterative scarring leading to a revision surgery in only 5 patients (3.3%) [1].

Retrobulbar hemorrhage may occur after peribulbar injection of local anesthetics [7], rather than from surgery itself.

8.4 Recommendations to Prevent Complications and How to Treat Them

Since our endoscopic technique includes the creation of an inferiorly based mucosal flap which is put back at the end of the procedure covering the lateral aspect of the nose, the incidence of ecchymosis of the cheek could considerably be reduced in our hands. Cheek ecchymosis in the immediate postoperative period should be treated with ice packs. Heparin ointment may help in its reabsorption.

Patients are carefully instructed not to blow their nose or to sneeze with their mouth open for a safety period of about 10 days after surgery in order to prevent increased pressure within the nose; thus, emphysemas of the soft tissues, including the orbit, are avoided. If an emphysema of the cheek occurs, it is important to prevent its growth by prohibiting further nose blowing. In orbital emphysemas we regularly prescribe antibiotics, whereas in cheek emphysema it depends on the presence or not of infection (pus) in the lacrimal sac [8].

No tension should be applied to the silicone stent when it is fixed on the nose. Patients should be able to open the eye without limitations. Knotting the stent inside the nose does not at all prevent displacement of the stent, the catheter then protruding onto the cornea. Fully displaced or extruded stents do not need to be replaced, as the functional outcome does not depend on the stenting. As for the outcome, silicone stenting is not necessary in conventional endonasal DCR except in the case of presaccal stenosis [10]; however, it may help during the follow-up when removal of fibrin, blood clots, and crusts is performed endoscopically.

Closure of the newly created ostium may happen when bone has been left near the common canaliculus, serving as a scaffold for obliterative scarring. Intraoperative removal of the bone surrounding the common canaliculus, at the superior third of the lacrimal sac, prevents the bone to act as a scaffold for fibroblast ingrowth, and thus, obliterative scarring. Once the drainage is closed, leading to recurrent epiphora, it probably may need a revision surgery. Topical use of mitomycin C (MMC) is said to modulate the scarring process, preventing the occlusion [11]. Application of artificial tears (eyedrops) containing steroids and antibiotics help to maintain the patency. In our hands, the best prevention of obliterative scarring consists in creating a large ostium at the level of the common canaliculus.

Burning of the skin can be avoided with a long hand piece or a protected drill and using the burr only until the lacrimal sac is partially exposed.

Displacement or loss of the silicone tube can be prevented by fixing both ends of the probe to the dorsum of the nose and allowing the eyelids to open sufficiently. In order to avoid pulling internal knotting is recommended in children only [12].

After more than 600 cases of endoscopic DCR we can recommend to withdraw the silicone catheter after a period of about 2–3 weeks, which is a tolerable period for patients. Functional results do not depend on the silicone probe, but rather on the exposure of the common canaliculus; however, the probe facilitates the draining of tears and of eyedrops, as well as endoscopic follow-ups. Granulation tissue at the internal ostium require an early removal of the probe, which probably acts as a foreign body, and subsequent treatment consisting of nasal douching with saline plus topical steroids.

Minor synechiae can be avoided preserving mucosa of the middle turbinate. Middle turbinates tilting laterally may be trimmed.

Reference

1. Bernal Sprekelsen M, Tomás Barberán M. Endoscopic dacriocystorhinostomy. Surgical technique and results. Laryngoscope 1996; 106:187–189

2. Fayet B, Racy E, Assouline M.Complications of standardized endonasal dacryocystorhinostomy with unciformectomy. Ophthalmology 2004; 111:837–845
3. Cokkeser Y, Evereklioglu C, Tercan M, Hepsen IF. Hammer–chisel technique in endoscopic dacryocystorhinostomy. Ann Otol Rhinol Laryngol 2003; 112:444–449
4. Massegur H, Trias E, Adema JM. Endoscopic dacryocystorhinostomy: modified technique. Otolaryngol Head Neck Surg 2004; 130:39–46
5. Dolman PJ.Comparison of external dacryocystorhinostomy with nonlaser endonasal dacryocystorhinostomy. Ophthalmology 2003; 110:78–84
6. Zilelioglu G, Tekeli O, Ugurba SH, Akiner M, Akturk T, Anadolu Y. Results of endoscopic endonasal non-laser dacryocystorhinostomy. Doc Ophthalmol 2002; 105:57–62
7. McNab AA, Simmie RJ. Effectiveness of local anaesthesia for external dacryocystorhinostomy. Clin Experiment Ophthalmol 2002; 30:270–272
8. Bernal Sprekelsen M. La dacriocistorrinostomía endoscópica. Otorrinolaringológica (Arg.) 1995; 4:61–68
9. Bernal Sprekelsen M. Die endoskopische Tränenwegschirurgie. Laryngo-Rhino-Otol 1998; 11: 650–651
10. Keerl R, Weber R. Dacryocystorhinostomy: state of the art, indications, results. Laryngorhinootologie 2004; 83:40–50
11. Ahmad SS, Untoo RA. Results of intraoperative mitomycin C application in dacryocystorhinostomy. J Sci 2002; 4:27–31
12. Bernal Sprekelsen M, Massegur H, Tomas M. Endoscopic sinus surgery in children. Rev Laryngol Otol Rhinol 2003; 124:145–150

Chapter 9

Nasolacrimal System Injuries

D.A. Della Rocca, S. Ahmad, P. Preechawi, S.D. Schaefer and R.C. Della Rocca

9

Core Messages

- Damage to the lacrimal drainage system can cause telecanthus, globe displacement, epiphora, or obstructive dacryocystitis. It can affect patients both functionally and cosmetically.
- It is essential to carefully check for any associated injuries such as neurological, thoracic, and abdominal trauma when significant facial trauma occurs.
- An appropriate ocular examination and visual assessment should be performed.
- A facial CT scan is required in any patients suspected of having nasoethmoid injuries.
- Early one-stage repair is recommended. It consists of exposure of all fracture fragments and precise anatomic rigid fixation, immediate bone grafting, if needed, and definitive soft tissue management.

Contents

9.1 Introduction

This chapter describes the evaluation and treatment of injuries to nasolacrimal system. Isolated nasoethmoid-orbital injuries are common. The most frequent causes are high-energy traumas, such as motor vehicle accidents [1, 2], by an impact force applied to the upper portion of the bridge of nose [3]. Often, a closed fracture is transformed into a compound one by laceration, avulsion, or bursting of the soft tissue of the naso-orbital area [4].

The patient with nasolacrimal injuries may present with significant concurrent facial wounds, and multiple system injuries. Such patients must be rapidly evaluated and stabilized. The American College of Surgeons (ACS) has developed an Advanced Trauma Life Support (ATLS) protocol to guide one through the four steps of primary survey, resuscitation, secondary survey, and definitive treatment. The primary survey focuses on the ABCs, i.e., airway, breathing, and circulation. In the facial injury patient, airway evaluation must include assessment of the patency of the upper aerodigestive track followed by assessing breathing effort. Possible etiologies of impaired airway in these patients are facial fractures, foreign bodies, laryngeal injuries, and expanding hematomas. Impaired breathing may reflect neurological injuries sustained during the facial injury to direct trauma to the thorax. Poor perfusion of the head and neck, or more distal sites, suggests shock. Shock may be divided into neurological, cardiac, septic, and hypovolemic etiologies. Neurological and hypovolemic shock are the most common forms of shock in the patient with trauma confined to the head. Resuscitation begins with establishing a patent airway. This may be as simple as removing foreign bodies, blood, or mucus to intubation or surgical establishment of an airway. As the patient with head injuries may also have cervical spine trauma, the neck should be stabilized by sand bags, and manipulation of the head may be minimized until this site is further evaluated. Following the critical steps of the primary survey, the secondary survey should be performed. This part of the ATLS protocol recapitulates the *ABC* of the primary survey, and also includes the detailing the disability (D) and exposure or examination (E) to better define the injury. Depending on the findings in the primary survey, attention is now focused on such areas as the definitive neurological examination; cervical spine, chest, or abdominal radiography; and careful examination of the imaging and angiography. Following stabilization of the patient, and appropriate definitive management of more severe injuries, the patient can now enter the stage of definitive treatment of the nasolacrimal injury.

Anatomical landmarks in this area are helpful. They include the medial orbital wall, the medial canthal tendon, the eyelids, and the lacrimal drainage system. Damage to the structures can cause telecanthus, globe displacement, epiphora, or obstructive dacryocystitis [1–18]. It can affect patients both functionally and cosmetically. A systemic treatment approach towards diagnosis and treatment is necessary.

9.2 Anatomical Considerations

9.2.1 Osteology

Regarding anatomical considerations [19–21], the bony aspects of the nasolacrimal excretory system exist at the medial wall of the anterior orbit and extend to the lateral wall of the nasal wall. The lacrimal fossa of the orbit is composed of the maxilla anteriorly and the lacrimal bone posteriorly. The lacrimal fossa is a shallow depression bounded by the anterior lacrimal crest and the posterior lacrimal crest. The maxillolacrimal suture runs vertically within the lacrimal fossa. At the inferior aspect of the depression is the ostium of the nasolacrimal duct which extends through the maxillary bone and exits under the inferior turbinate of the nose (Fig. 9.1).

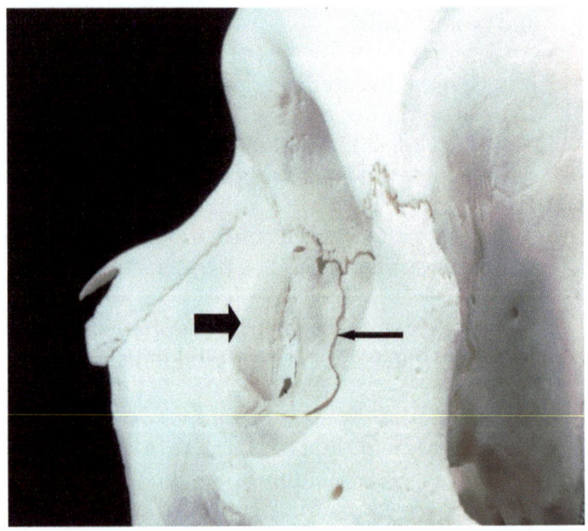

Fig. 9.1. The fossa for the lacrimal sac lies anterior to the lamina papyracea of the medial orbital wall. It is bordered by a rounded anterior lacrimal crest (*thick arrow*) and a sharply defined posterior lacrimal crest (*thin arrow*). Direct mid facial trauma can cause displacement of the lacrimal sac associated with fractures

9.2.2 Soft Tissue

The described osteology serves as a scaffolding for both the suspensory elements of the eyelid and the lacrimal excretory system. The anterior lamellae of the eyelid consists largely of skin and the orbicularis muscle. The orbicularis, which acts as the protractor of the eyelids, has a complex arrangement to where it originates at the medial wall. At this origin, the preseptal orbicularis is divided into a superficial head and deep (Jones muscle) head. The superficial head extends from the anterior rim of the medial canthal tendon which itself originates from the anterior lacrimal crest. The deep head of the preseptal orbicularis originates at the lacrimal sac and its connective tissues.

The pretarsal orbicularis is adherent to the tarsus of the upper and lower eyelids. This is also split into superficial and deep (Horner's tensor tarsi muscle) segments. The deep head extends from 4 mm posterior to the posterior lacrimal crest. This muscle's posterior orientation allows for proper contour of the medial canthus and appropriate apposition of the eyelids to the medial aspect of the eye globe. The superficial horns of the pretarsal orbicularis inserts on the anterior edge of medial canthal tendon.

The complex arrangements of the muscles allows for a lacrimal pump of positive and negative pressures which helps move the tears within the palpebral fissures through the lacrimal excretory system. Bony and soft tissue traumatic injury to these structures may eliminate "lacrimal pump" physiology.

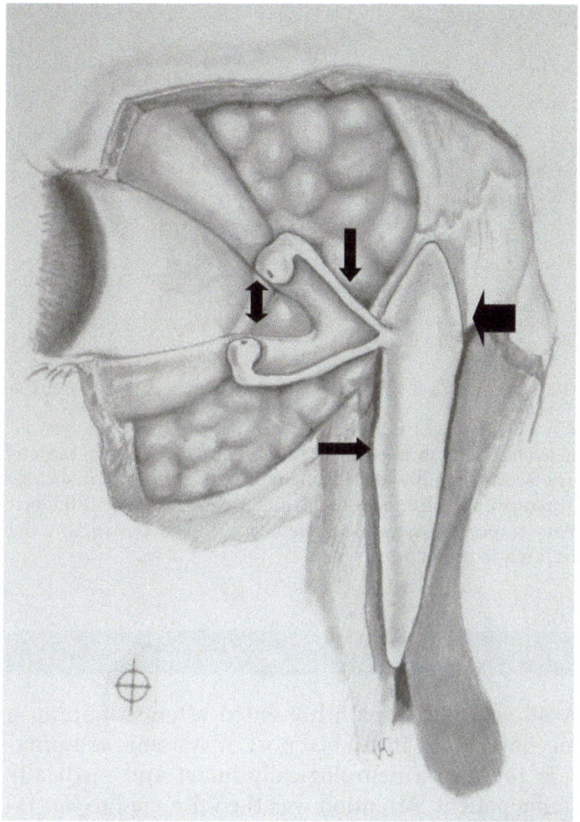

Fig. 9.2. The lacrimal drainage system includes the punctum (*double arrow*), the canaliculi (*vertical down arrow*) , lacrimal sac (*thick arrow*), and naso-lacrimal duct (*left arrow*). Soft tissue lacerations may include distal and proximal canaliculi while bony trauma can affect the lacrimal sac and the naso-lacrimal duct

9.2.3 Lacrimal Excretory System

The lacrimal system begins at the lacrimal punctum which starts at the myocutaneous junction of the medial aspect of the lid margin of upper and lower eyelids. The punctum are surrounded by a fibrous ring called the lacrimal papilla which is in turn surrounded by the pretarsal orbicularis.

The canaliculi extends form the punctum to the lacrimal sac. The caniliculus initially has a vertical path of 2 mm followed by a medial extension toward the lacrimal sac. The medial extension (8–10 mm) follows a horizontal pathway hugging the contour of the eyelid margin. As the canaliculi approach the lacrimal sac, they tend to combine to form the common canaliculus. This final pathway enters the lateral wall of the lacrimal sac slightly above the vertical midpoint of the sac.

The lacrimal sac lies within the bony depression of the medial orbital wall, called the fossa of the lacrimal sac. The sack measures 12 mm in height, 4–6 mm in depth, and 2 mm in width. The shape is pisciform with a narrower top and wider lower portion. The sack is bound by the fossa medially, the medial canthal tendon superiorly, and muscle and orbital septum inferomedially.

The lacrimal duct measures 3–4 mm in diameter and extends inferiorly 12.5 mm vertically. The upper part of the duct runs through the maxilla while the inferior part runs within the nasal mucosa of the lateral nasal wall. The mucosa lining of the duct exits at the lateral wall of the nasal passage of the inferior meatus. The flap of mucosa at this exit is referred to as the Valve of Hasner. Both the lacrimal sac and duct can be injured with facial and nasojugal lacerations in addition to being obstructed with orbit and maxillary fractures (Fig. 9.2)

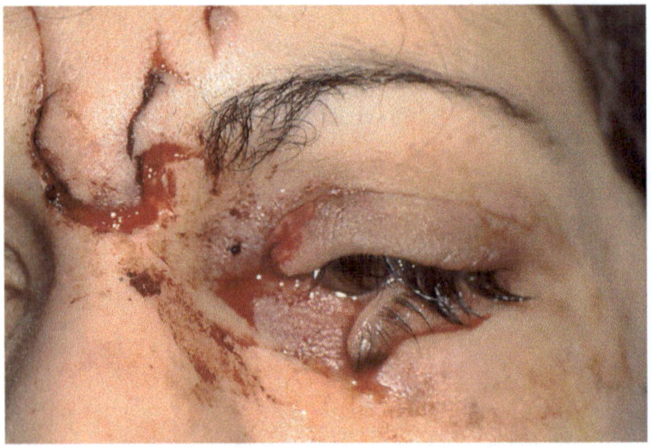

Fig. 9.3. A 46-year-old patient with large glabellar laceration, an avulsed laceration of the upper and lower eyelids, and extensive laceration of the distal canaliculi and common canalicular structures. Establishment of the integrity of the globe is the primary responsibility of the surgeon prior to reconstructing the eyelids and the lacrimal system

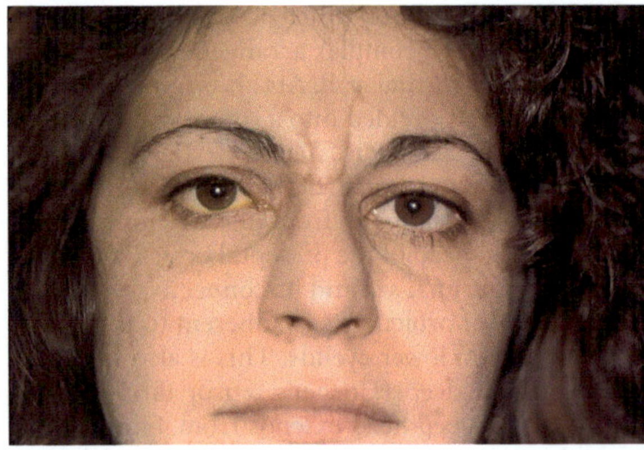

Fig. 9.4. The patient is seen 3 month post-repair. The eyelid and canthus are in good position and the silastic tube will remain for 2 more months. Further glabellar surgery is planned including thinning and repositioning of the flap

9.3 Case History

A 46-year-old woman presented after sustaining a mechanical fall into a bed post. A systemic examination revealed a neurologically intact and medically stable patient. Attention was then directed to her facial injuries. Clinical assessment revealed a large avulsed laceration extending from the glabellar area down to the bridge of the nose, a 50% avulsed laceration of the lower eyelid originating from the medial canthal area and a distal upper eyelid canthal laceration with injury to the canalicular system. A traction test confirmed a disrupted medial canthal tendon. Palpation over the bones demonstrated no bony crepitus or clicks. Ophthalmic examination showed 20/20 vision OU, no pupillary deficits, and a normal fundoscopic examination. A facial computed tomography (CT) scan was negative for any nasoethmoidal fractures (Fig. 9.3).

Surgical intervention was carried out under general anesthesia. Exploration of the lacerations confirmed the preoperative assessment. Repair of both upper and lower eyelid lacerations was performed after bicanalicular silicone intubation and repair of the upper canalicular laceration. The medial canthal avulsion was re-approximated using deep sutures and bolsters and completing medial canthopexy. Finally, the glabellar laceration was repaired (Fig. 9.4).

9.4 Diagnosis and Clinical Assessment

The incidence of facial injuries is high because the face is in an exposed position [14]. A study [22] confirmed that the nasal area is the weakest portion of the facial skeleton and fractures may occur with a blunt impact load of 35–80 g. With trauma the maintenance of a patent airway in severe naso-orbital trauma is paramount. It is essential to carefully check for any associated injuries such as neurological, thoracic, and abdominal trauma when significant facial trauma occurs.

The physical examination should begin with an assessment of the soft tissues. Swelling, ecchymoses, and lacerations are noted. Lacerations in the medial canthal region should be assessed to determine the integrity of the lacrimal drainage system and medial canthal tendon. A disruption of the medial canthal tendon can be assessed by a "traction test" [2, 9]. It is done by grasping the edge of the lower eyelid or upper eyelid laterally and pulling against the medial attachment. If the eyelid margin does not become taut and bowstring, or you feel asymmetry in the two sides, then with avulsion the medial portion of the tendon has likely been disrupted.

The other important structures in this area are the upper and lower canaliculi. Firstly, inspection of the lacrimal and canthal area is completed. A cotton-tipped swab is used to gently palpate eyelid tissue.

This can help define the location and extent of the injury. In addition, an accurate evaluation of the lacrimal drainage effectiveness, irrigation, and probing should be performed. The presence of canalicular laceration requires silicone intubation and repair of the laceration. The distal lacrimal system, including the lacrimal sac and the nasolacrimal duct, tends not to be affected by trauma because they are well protected by the bony structures.

Inspection and physical examination of the patients with nasoethmoid–orbital injuries can help predict the sites and extent of fractures prior to radiographical studies. The palpation over the bones onto the medial canthal tendon attachment will give good information [23]. This palpation may demonstrate bony crepitus or clicks depending on the degree of instability. The width and the symmetry of the medial canthi should be assessed for telecanthus. The normal intercanthal width ranges from 30 to 35 mm in whites [9, 24, 25], or half of interpupillary distance [9, 26], which is a more reliable guide. The third guide which might be used for the intercanthal width is equal to the alar–alar width at the base of the nose. The other obvious sign is saddle nose deformity which means loss of nasal skeletal support. Furthermore, typically, the medial aspect of the palpebral fissure may lose its sharpness and become rounded and slack with varying degrees of downward and outward displacement.

An ocular examination should be performed. Injuries in this area may be associated with ophthalmic emergency and problems such as ruptured globe or traumatic optic neuropathy especially when the principle fracture or displacement involves bones of the apex of the orbit [27–30]. There is no accurate incidence of ocular injuries associated with nasolacrimal injuries, because many studies vary in the level of ophthalmic evaluation; however, a study by Holt et al. [31] found 59% of nasal fractures showed concomitant eye injuries and 76% of midfacial fractures were associated with eye injuries. For the severity of ocular injuries, 79% were temporary or minor, and 18% were serious, defined as sustained visual loss or adnexal sequelae requiring subsequent reconstructive measures; 3% resulted in blindness. Therefore, an initial ocular evaluation in mid-facial fractures is necessary [32–34]. Useful guidelines are as follows:

1. Develop a brief historical profile of pre-injury vision, current subjective visual status, current eye disease, and previous intraocular surgery.
2. Obtain an objective baseline visual acuity, examine the pupils and afferent papillary defect (APD), eyelids, anterior segment, posterior segment, and ocular motility.
3. Evaluate the above findings to determine if ophthalmic consultation is needed.

In conclusion, patients with nasoethmoid–orbital injuries are evaluated in three ways. The bony involvement, such as nasoethmoid fracture or nasolacrimal, naso-orbital fractures, or complex fractures, should be considered. The soft tissue injuries are especially concerned in medial canthal tendon area and lacrimal drainage system which includes canaliculi and lacrimal sac. The third part is appropriate ocular examination and visual assessment.

A facial CT scan is required in any patients suspected of having nasoethmoid injuries. Axial and coronal images, spaced at 1.5 mm, are most effective in evaluating and classifying nasoethmoid–orbital fractures [35]. The CT scans not only define the presence and extent of the fractures, but additionally can show direct injury to the lacrimal sac and lacrimal duct.

9.5 General Principles

Management for nasoethmoid orbital injuries can be divided into two parts, bony fracture and soft tissue injuries which are divided into two subgroups, medial canthal tendon injuries, and lacrimal drainage system injuries.

Management of lacrimal drainage system injuries and medial canthal tendon injuries include the following [16]:

1. Early one-stage repair
2. Exposure of all fracture fragments
3. Precise anatomic rigid fixation
4. Immediate bone grafting, if needed
5. Definitive soft tissue management

Using these principles most late functional and aesthetic sequelae have been diminished or eliminated. The precise concept of management for these fractures is to do as much as possible at the first time [36]. It is unusual for the medial canthal tendon to be directly injured in this type of trauma (blunt trauma) [9] and, because of that repositioning of the bony complex, the proper intercanthal relationship should be adequately restored [37–40].

The management of fractures in this area, when extensive, is completed utilizing open reduction, rigid osteological fixation, and plate implants as required [3, 5, 9, 11, 16, 36].

The lacrimal system is not frequently injured in nasolacrimal injuries in the absence of medial canthal avulsion or obvious lacrimal system transection [11, 13]. The incidence of late lacrimal obstruction requiring dacryocystorhinostomy was 5–10% following acute fracture management [43].

The indications for surgery in a nasolacrimal trauma are those outlined above. Restoration of pre-injury facial aesthetics and function is the goal of treatment. Since these injuries are usually associated with significant cosmetic and functional sequelae, expeditious restoration of injuries and function prevents latent cosmetic and functional deficits. Longer-term follow-up allows the surgeon to assess for both early and late sequelae of injuries.

Definitive treatment of nasolacrimal injuries should be deferred until the patient has been stabilized regarding any concomitant, compromising, or life-threatening trauma. During this time, systemic deficits can be corrected while giving the surgeon time for an accurate assessment prior to the operative procedure. As with any operative procedure, the risks of general anesthesia and the stresses of surgery must be weighed against medical contraindications. Ocular contraindications include optic nerve injury and globe injury (e.g., hyphema, rupture, laceration). These injuries should be addressed and stabilized prior to surgical intervention, since osseous manipulation may exacerbate damage to the eye. Some injuries may not need correction, provided that the patient is satisfied with the appearance and function.

9.6 Management

While proper instrumentation is an essential element to the successful undertaking of surgical repair of nasolacrimal injuries, strict adherence to several basic surgical principles is more important. Intimate knowledge of anatomy, adequate anesthesia, excellent exposure of operative site, sufficient hemostasis, and proper wound closure will ultimately impact greater on the results than choice of manufacturer of instruments. One must also pay special attention to lighting, suction, and instruments.

Surgical vision aids include telescopic loops with magnification from 2.5–3.5 times with an adequate field of view and comfortable working distance. The operating microscope may also have a role in certain procedures. Illumination of the surgical field is key; preferably, the operating room should have two ceiling-mounted lamps to minimize shadowing of the field. Head-mounted fiberoptic lamps also very useful.

The basic lacrimal irrigation set should include punctal dilators, Bowman probes, a lacrimal irrigation cannula, and a syringe filled with balanced salt solution (BSS).

Prior to probing, nasal packing should be performed. A basic nasal packing set should include Codman sponges (cotton strips 1×7.5 cm) soaked in 0.25 or 0.5% phenylephrine, nasal specula, and Gruenwald (Jansen) forceps. A fiberoptic headlight may be used to illuminate and aid in the insertion the cotton pledgets into the nasal cavity. An endoscope may also aid in visualization of the nasal cavity.

A number of manufacturers produce lacrimal intubation systems (Jed-Med, Ritleng, FCI company). The authors prefer the Crawford intubation system manufactured by Jed-Med. This consists of a pair of flexible stainless steel olive-tipped intubation rods that are approximately #000 to #0000 in size and are attached to a silastic tube. The small tip size allows for easy passage through the upper and or lower puncta. The system also has a retrieval hook that is used to engage the olive tips when the tubes are externalized in the nares.

9.7 Anesthesia

The choice of anesthesia depends on several factors. Treatment in children must be performed under general anesthesia. For most adults, treatment can be performed with monitored anesthesia with intravenous sedation. Because of the difficult anatomy of the nose, especially in the setting of extensive nasoethmoidal orbital trauma or more extensive injuries, general anesthesia may be the preferred anesthetic approach. The surgeon's familiarity with the technique is also important, so that abundant bleeding is avoided under local anesthesia. Otherwise, in experienced hands, monitored anesthesia care (MAC) can be offered to adults and surgery can be performed on a day-surgery outpatient basis.

Local anesthesia has some advantages in preference to regional anesthesia for its hemostatic properties. The area of the lacrimal sac and both the superior and inferior medial aspects of the injured eyelid are first infiltrated with dilute anesthetic solution consisting of nine parts saline and one part 2% lidocaine (Xylocaine) with epinephrine 1:100,000 (in adults) or 0.5% lidocaine with 1:200,000 epinephrine (in children). The dilute anesthetic is less painful. Alternatively, 2% lidocaine with epinephrine can be mixed with bicarbonate in a 9-to-1 ratio. For maximum hemostasis, the anesthetic solution should be prepared "fresh" by adding 0.3 ml of epinephrine 1:1000 to a 30-ml bottle of 2% lidocaine and administered 10 min prior to the procedure. Epinephrine is not used if the patient has a history of coronary artery disease.

The sensation to the nose derives from the infratrochlear, infraorbital, supratrochlear, and anterior ethmoidal nerves. The base of the nose at the anterior septum, the nasal root, dorsum, lateral nasal walls, along with the middle turbinate, is infiltrated with 1–2% lidocaine with 1:100,000 epinephrine. This field block is more effective than targeted nerve blocks. Local hemostasis and anesthesia are augmented with nasal vasoconstrictors, such as phenylephrine soaked cottonoids. This may be preceded by topical decongestion and anesthesia (e.g., oxymetazoline, Cetacaine) to aid in more comfortable introduction of the pledgets. The physician must wait an adequate period (approximately 15–20 min) to allow the anesthesia and vasoconstriction to be effective.

The benefits of general anesthesia in orbital surgery and more complicated procedures are many: Firstly, it provides deep orbital anesthesia, especially during osteotomy procedures and other bone work, which is difficult to achieve with regional blockade. Secondly, it allows for monitoring of blood pressure and heart rate. It provides a relative systemic hypotension, which is helpful in reducing bleeding during orbital surgery. Thirdly, the necessary volume of injectable anesthetic agent is reduced, limiting the risk of systemic toxicity.

General anesthesia can be safely administered to the ambulatory patient; however, because of the great effect on cardiovascular and respiratory systems, emphasis is placed on the preoperative evaluation. Preexisting medical conditions need to be treated preoperatively to ensure that the patient is in the best possible health prior to surgery. Of particular importance is a recent history of myocardial infarction, hypertension, cardiac arrhythmia, and chronic obstructive pulmonary disease, and diabetes. General anesthesia may be inappropriate for patients with poor systemic health, particularly those with advanced cardiovascular or pulmonary disease.

9.8 Canalicular Laceration

Lacerations to the canaliculus should be treated primarily while injury to the lacrimal sac or nasolacrimal duct can be operated on later [44], because there is a chance of spontaneous improvement. Studies of canalicular lacerations by experiments and retrospective analysis [45] suggest that canalicular portion of the eyelid is particularly vulnerable to shearing, avulsion, and stretching forces. Canalicular lacerations may occur by direct lacerations of the canaliculus or from diffuse or indirect injury. If the inferior canaliculus is lacerated, bicanalicular silicone intubation is preferred over monocanalicular intubation. In addition to being more stable within the lacrimal system, bicanalicular intubation of the lacrimal system is particularly effective in defining the medial canthus and commissure when treating medial canthal and eyelid avulsions.

9.9 Operative Technique

Repair of the canalicular system is optimally done under general anesthesia. Microsurgical repair by surgical loops or operating microscope is necessary [6, 46]. Before starting repair, it is important to constrict the nasal mucosa with oxymethazoline or 0.25% phenylephrine on cotton pledgets placed inferiorly to the inferior turbinate. This will shrink the inferior turbinate and improve visualization. Following this, injection with 2% lidocaine with epinephrine 1:100,000 is done followed by repacking of the inferior meatus with the soaked cotton pledgets.

The punctal dilator is used to enlarge punctum and the lacrimal probe is used to navigate the proximal canaliculus until the cut canaliculus is identified laterally. Canalicular injuries should be repaired within 24–48 h after injuries [6, 46], because the medial cut edge of canaliculus becomes progressively more difficult to identify as fibrin and granulation deposition occurs. The medial cut edge of canaliculus is identified successfully by direct inspection. The cut canaliculus is identified as white mucosal tissue with wall and lumens. Deliberate inspection with gentle traction of the crowded tissue is often necessary. If discovery of the lumen remains difficult, injection of air into the uncut canaliculus while observing the medial cut area submerged in saline may uncover its location with the appearance of air bubbles [47–49]. Also, skin hooks and silk traction sutures can be used to retract the medial eyelid tissue as necessary.

After identification of the medial cut edge of the canaliculus, a Crawford tube is used to intubate the distal canaliculus and the lacrimal sac and duct. Following this, a metallic probe attached to silicone tubing is insinuated into the proximal canaliculus, distal canaliculus, and then the lacrimal sack and duct. It is necessary to orient the probe to follow the anatomical course of the lacrimal system. Because visualization of the distal canaliculus is easily lost, it is useful to keep the Crawford tube in place until the moment of intubation with the silicone tubing. The hook or grooved dissector is used to deliver the probe from beneath the inferior turbinate and out the nostril. When a bicanilicular system is used, the opposite canilicular system is insinuated in a similar way and retrieved through the nares.

The canaliculus can be approximated by two to three absorbable 8-0 sutures placed in the mucosal wall of cut canaliculus in order to achieve an end-to-end anastomosis of the tube [50, 51]. Some authors [52, 53] used single stitch repairs with 7-0 vicryl horizontal mattress sutures, which passed in the plane directly anterior to the canaliculus. The results [52] are excellent, although 4% still have epiphora and 13% still have delay outflow with dye disappearance test.

With compete avulsion of the medial canthus from its origin at the anterior lacrimal crest, reapproximation can be done with a double armed 4-0 silk suture. This suture should be placed through the lateral wound edge with a substantial bite followed by a deep medial bite which would ideally include periostium of the anterior lacrimal crest. The sutures should be tied over the skin using bolsters of foam or rubber.

With bicanilicular intubation, the distal tube ends are joined with five single throws of the silicone suture. The silicone should have enough tension on it to recess at least 1.5 cm into the nares after they are tied and released.

If the eyelid margin lacerated, 6-0 silk suture is placed through three layers, tarsus to tarsus via meibomian orifice, gray line, and lash line. These marginal sutures should be reflected away from the globe and tied to skin (Figs. 9.5–9.13).

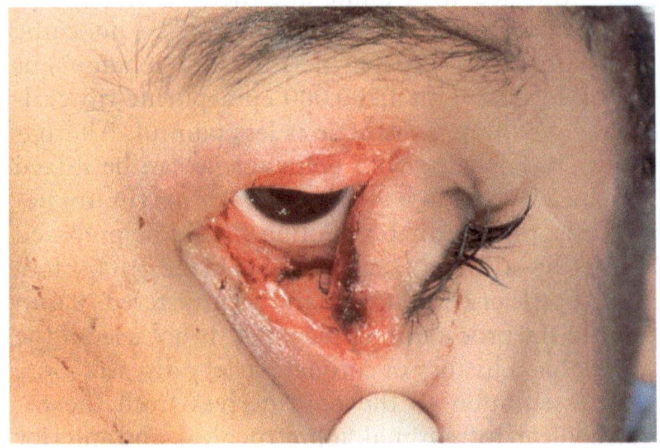

Fig. 9.5. A patient with complete avulsion of the upper and lower eyelids with canalicular injury. In the upper eyelid it is important to identify and repair the levator muscle that has been lacerated. The repair is done in three layers (the conjunctiva, the levator, and the skin). It is difficult in these cases to identify the distal lacerated common canaliculi. The use of the surgical microscope and painstaking repair is required to affect good result

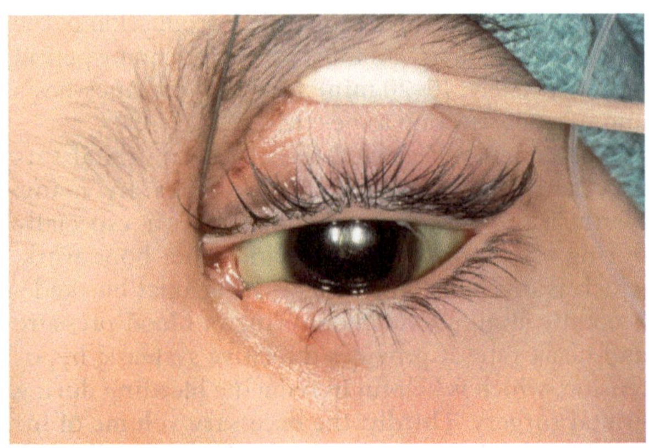

Fig. 9.6. Same patient. After punctal dilation, the Bowman probe 0-0 is passed through the upper canaliculus, through the naso lacrimal system, through the valve of Hasner, and then into the nose. The direction of the probe will be helpful when the Crawford intubation is done

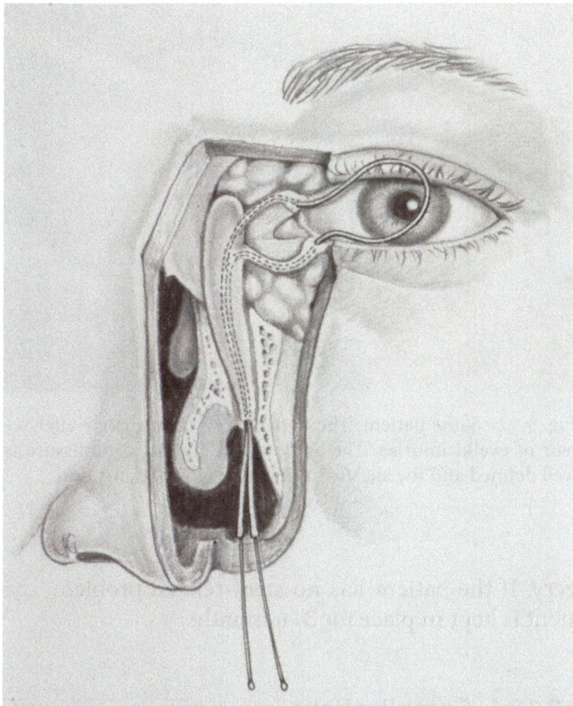

Fig. 9.7. Same patient. One olive-piped rod of the double armed silastic tube is placed through the upper canalicular system while the other is placed through the lower canalicular system. Each rod is retrieved in the nares, leaving a loop of tubing between the upper and lower punctum (demonstrated here with Crawford tube system)

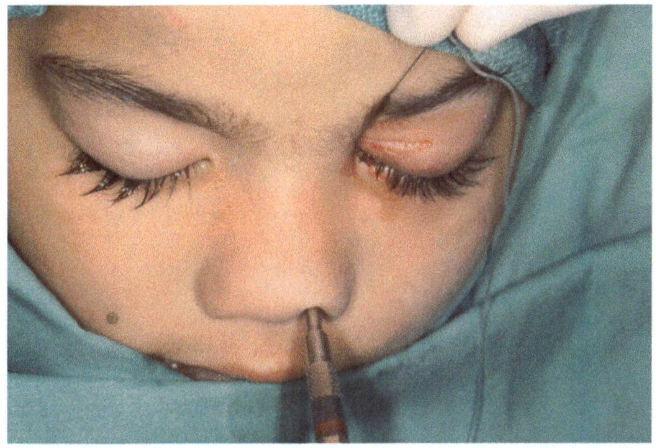

Fig. 9.8. Same patient. The Crawford probe and tube is passed into and through the lacrimal system. After the Bowman probe has helped to define the direction of the angle into the nose. The Freer elevator is used to palpate the end of the probe in preparation for the retrieval of the Crawford tube

In conclusion, the principal techniques for repair canalicular laceration are:

1. Reanastomosis of the cut edge
2. Endocanalicular support with silicone tube
3. Use of direct catheterization if possible, or with an inexperienced surgeon, to avoid uninjured canaliculus injury

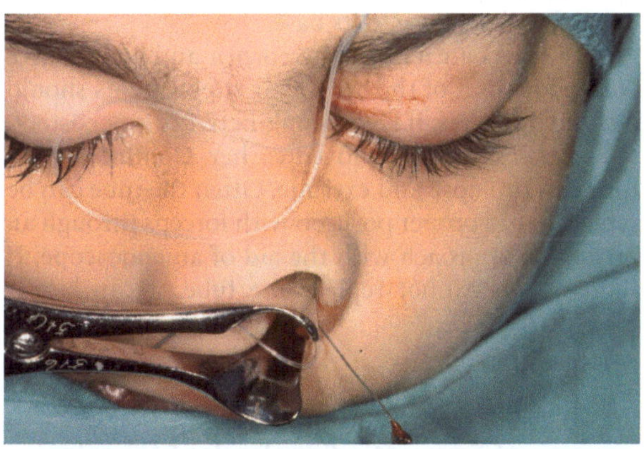

Fig. 9.9. Same patient. An olive-tipped probe has been grasped by the hook to complete the bicanalicular intubation. Shrinkage of the inferior turbinate with the use of a vasoconstrictor is helpful in the identification of the Crawford probe prior to grasping it. Nasal endoscopy can be quite helpful in this step

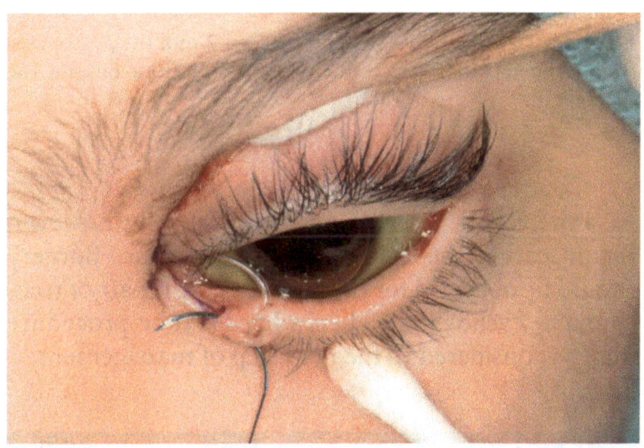

Fig. 9.10. Same patient. After intubation has been completed, the tissues are brought into position. Repair of the canalicula and eyelid laceration is then completed. A 4-0 double-armed silk suture is passed anterior and superior to the tube over a sponge bolster

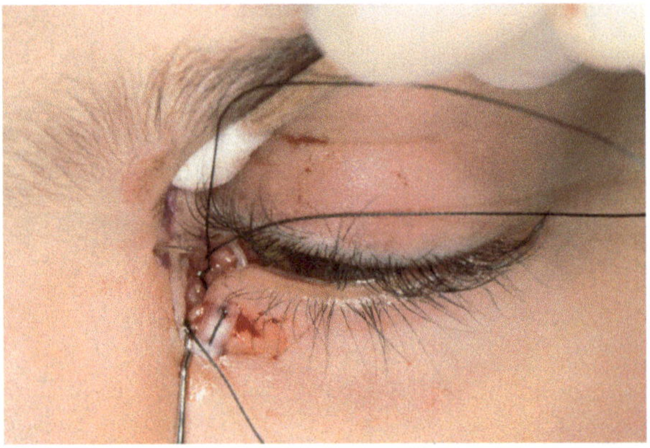

Fig. 9.11. Same patient. A double-armed needle is passed anterior to the medial canthal tendon in a superior medial direction. The double arm suture is passed through a similar bolster and tied after the lacerated eyelid margins are repaired

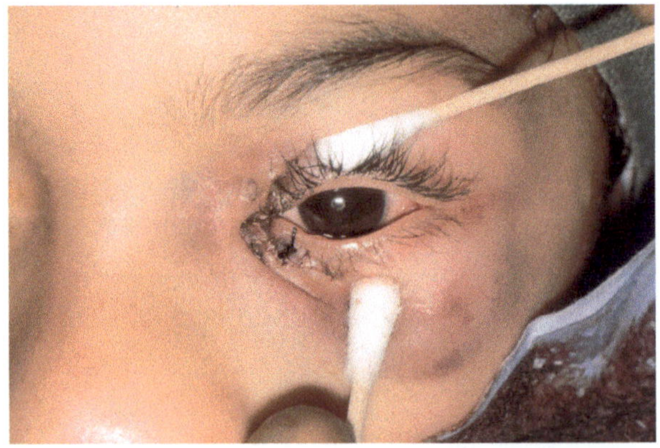

Fig. 9.12. Same patient. The patient seen immediately after repair of eyelid injuries. The angle of the medial commissure is well defined and the silastic intubation is in good position

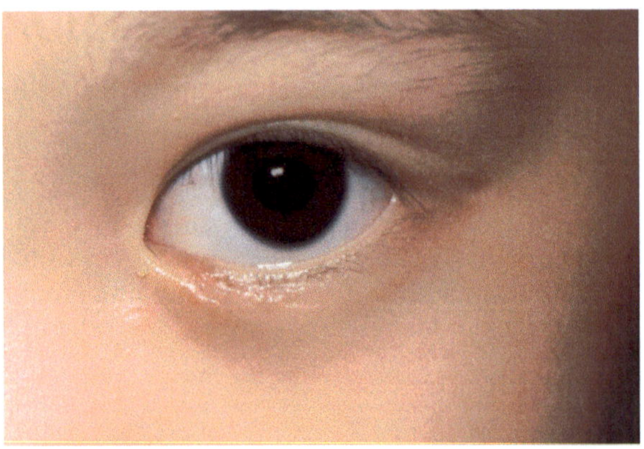

Fig. 9.13. Same patient. The patient seen 2 months postoperatively. The repair is successful with no epiphora despite the severe injury

In some very severe and extensive injuries, however, repair cannot be achieved the first time. Surgery should be obtained for the best possible repair of fracture and eyelids [54]. Then a bypass tube procedure may be considered in the next step of management.

9.10 Postoperative Care

Following silicone tube intubation, the patient is given steroid–antibiotic eye drops four times a day for 1 week. The patient is reevaluated at 1 week after surgery. If the patient has no stent-related problem, the stent is kept in place for 3–6 months.

9.10.1 Complications of Silicone Tube Intubation

Generally, the silicone rods are well tolerated; however, if the tube is tied too tightly, or the lacrimal papilla is compromised, "cheese wiring" through the puncta and canaliculi may occur, necessitating the removal of the tube. A pyogenic granuloma may develop near the punctum in some cases and should be excised with cautery to its base.

The tube can irritate the cornea and conjunctiva with adduction of the eyes. Tear supplements should be used; however, if keratoconjunctivitis is persistent, the tube should be removed earlier. Commonly, the tube can prolapse and extrude. Often the tube can be replaced into proper position with forceps through an intranasal approach with the aid of an endoscope. If the surgeon cannot replace the tube, it can be removed.

9.10.2 Secondary Repair of Traumatic Canalicular Stenosis

If epiphora exists in patients with eyelid lacerations, one should suspect unidentified or undetected canalicular involvement. It is possible to repair at a later date by excising the scar and reanastomoses the normal lumen, followed by bicanalicular silicone intubation [50, 55]. A nasolacrimal probe is passed into the punctum and passed to the site of obstruction. The eyelid is incised at this location. The purpose is to identify the proximal and distal ends of the lacerated canaliculus. At this time bicanilicular intubation is completed, if possible.

9.10.3 Lacrimal Sac and Nasolacrimal Duct Injuries

The incidence of persistent nasolacrimal system obstruction requiring DCR ranged from 5 to 21% [13, 41, 42]. As previously mentioned, the management of lacrimal sac and nasolacrimal duct injuries should not be explored at the initial surgery if there is no obvious laceration [11, 14, 41–43]. The rationale is that it is difficult in adequate assessment and repair especially of the severe injury because of soft tissue edema and hemorrhage. Trauma to lacrimal pathways can produce temporary or permanent dysfunction. Temporary dysfunction is caused by lacrimal compression by posttraumatic edema. There were studies [41, 42] that showed spontaneous resolution of traumatic epiphora within 6 months after primary fracture repair. Persistent dysfunction is a result of direct causes such as detachment of the medial canthal ligament with subsequent sac compression and pumping failure.

Irrigation of the system during primary fracture reconstruction or early postoperative period is not helpful due to edema and inflammation of the nasolacrimal duct. We recommend better assessment 1–3 months after trauma when resolution of edema and soft tissue injuries permit the definitive evaluation. Using fluorescein dye instilled into inferior cul-de-sac then waiting 5 min to reevaluate, if dye still persists in cul-de-sac, it means that there is nasolacrimal duct obstruction. The other investigation that is useful for evaluating post-traumatic nasolacrimal duct obstruction is CT scan and dacryocystography (DCG) [56–60] or combined CT and DCG. The combination of CT and DCG will give the useful information of complexity of anatomical change after trauma and repair, identify location of the lacrimal sac, bony structure, plate and screw implantation, and nasal septum which help in planning surgery.

For obvious laceration of the lacrimal sac or nasolacrimal duct there are different techniques to perform. Some authors advise applying silicone tube from punctum through the lacrimal sac and nasolacrimal duct [14, 42], but only if this can be done easily. If any difficulty is encountered, the attempts should be curtailed to avoid damage to the canalicular system. Subsequent DCR surgery may be done, if necessary, when the healing process is complete, usually 6 months after injury [41].

9.10.4 Different DCR Technique in Post-traumatic Patients

In traumatic cases the surgical technique for DCR differs in several aspects from routine DCR [41, 42]:

1. The skin incision is somewhat lengthened.
2. An attempt to avoid cutting of orbicularis oculi muscle fibers to maintain lacrimal pump function previously compromised by injury.
3. Bone removal may require bone drilling because bone can be thicker from the inflammation or impacted from the trauma. Care must be taken to avoid perforating the nasal mucosa.
4. Delay secondary repair at least 5–6 months from primary repair and the subsequent DCR decreases friability of the sac and nasal mucosa.

Silicone intubation is utilized in all cases because of the presumed predisposition to inflammation after trauma.

9.10.5 Conjunctivodacryocystorhinostomy with Jones Tube Intubation

In some instances, common punctum reconstruction cannot be accomplished because of extensive scarring involving the lacrimal sac or displaced lacrimal bone. Conjunctivodacryocysorhinostomy (CDCR) requires the placement of a Jones tube or similar bypass stent from the caruncle region directly through the lateral nasal mucosal wall following a large osteotomy. Prior to surgery, the patient requires counseling on the need for personal care of the tube and possible revision of the tube position.

9

Reference

1. Epker BN. Open surgical management of naso-orbital-ethmoid facial fractures. Trans Int Conf Oral Surg 1973;4:323–329
2. Fedok FG. Comprehensive management of nasoethmoid-orbital injuries. J Craniomaxillofac Trauma 1995;1:36–48
3. Converse JM, Smith B. Naso-orbital fractures and traumatic deformities of the medial canthus. Plast Reconstr Surg 1966;38:147–162
4. Smith BC, Barr DR, Langham EJ. Complication of orbital fractures. N Y S J Med 1971;71:2407–2411
5. Stranc MF. Primary treatment of naso-ethmoid injuries with increased intercanthal distance.Br J Plast Surg 1970;23:8–25
6. Lindsey JT. Lacrimal duct injuries revisited: a retrospective review of six patients. Ann Plast Surg 2000;44:167–172
7. Ramselaar JM, van der Meulen JC, Bloem JJ. Naso-orbital fractures. Mod Probl Ophthal 1975;14:607–610
8. Smith B. Late bilateral naso-orbital fracture and dacryostenosis. Trans Am Acad Ophthalmol Otolaryngol 1972;76:1378–1379
9. Holt GR, Holt JE. Nasoethmoid complex injuries. Otolaryngol Clin N Am 1985;18:87–98
10. Harris GJ, Fuerste FH. Lacrimal intubation in the primary repair of midfacial fractures. Ophthalmology 1987;94:242–247
11. Leipziger LS, Manson PN. Nasoethmoid orbital fractures. Clin Plast Surg 1992;19:167–193
12. White MJ, Johnson PC, Heckler FR. Management of maxillofacial and neck soft tissue injuries. Clin Sports Med 1989;8:11–23
13. Stranc MF. The pattern of lacrimal injuries in naso-ethmoid fractures. Br J Plast Surg 1970;23:339–346
14. Gruss JS. Fronto-naso-orbital trauma. Clin Plast Surg 1982;9:577–589
15. Katowitz JA, Diamond G. Ophthalmic consideration in cranio-orbital surgery. Clin Plast Surg 1987;14:155–162
16. Rohrich RJ, Shewmake KB. Evolving concepts of craniomaxillofacial fracture management. Clin Plast Surg 1992;19:1–10
17. Spinelli HM, Forman DL. Current treatment of post-traumatic deformities. Clin Plast Surg 1997;24:519–530
18. Merville LC, Real JP. Fronto-orbital nasal dislocation. Scand J Plast Reconstr Surg 1980;15:287–297
19. Lemke BN, Della Rocca RC. The eyelids; medial canthal tendon: anatomy and surgery. Norwalk: Appleton and Lange, 1990:199–202
20. Shovlin JP, Lemke BN. Clinical eyelid anatomy. In: Bosniak S, ed. Principle and practice of ophthalmic plastic and reconstructive surgery, Philadelphia: Saunders, 1996:261–280
21. Nerad JA. Clinical anatomy. In: Nerad JA, ed. Oculoplastic surgery: the requisites in ophthalmology. St. Louis: Mosby, 2001:25–70
22. Swearingen JJ. Tolerances of the human face to crash impact. Federal Aviation Agency, Oklahoma City, 1965
23. Paskert JP, Manson PN. The bimanual examination for assessing instability in naso-orbitoethmoidal injuries. Plast Reconstr Surg 1989;83:165–167
24. Hansman CF. Growth of interorbital distance and skull thickness as observed in roentgenographic measurements. Radiology 1966;86:87–96
25. Freihofer HP. Inner intercanthal and interorbital distances. J Maxillofac Surg 1980;8:324–326
26. Collin JRO, Tyers AG. Preoperative evaluation. In: Collin JRO, Tyers AG, eds. Colour atlas of ophthalmic plastic surgery. Oxford: Butterworth-Heinemann, 2001:49–58
27. Hooper RS. Orbital complication of head injury. Br J Surg 1951;39:126
28. King AB, Walsh FB. Trauma to the head with particular reference to the ocular signs. Part I injuries involving the cranial nerves. Am J Ophthalmol 1949;32:191–205
29. Milauskas AT, Fueger GF. Serious ocular complication associated with blow-out fractures of the orbit. Am J Ophthalmol 1966;62:670–672
30. Miller GR, Tenzel RR. Ocular complication of mid-facial fractures. Plast Reconstr Surg 1967;39:37–42
31. Holt JE, Holt R, Blodgett JM. Ocular injuries sustained during blunt facial trauma. Ophthalmology 1983;90:14–18
32. Gossman MD, Roberts DM, Barr CC. Ophthalmic aspects of orbital injury: a comprehensive diagnostic and management approach. Clin Plast Surg 1992;19:71–85
33. Wessberg GA, Wolford LM, Zerdecki JW, et al. Ophthalmic consideration in maxillofacial trauma. Int J Oral Surg 1981;10:236–246
34. Pelletier CR, Jordan DR, Braga R, et al. Assessment of ocular trauma associated with head and neck injuries. J Trauma Injury Infect Crit Care 1998;44:350–354
35. Manson PN, Markowitz B, Mirvis S et al. Toward CT-based facial fracture treatment. Plast Reconstr Surg 1990;85:202
36. Lauritzen C, Lilja J, Vallfors B. The craniofacial approach to trauma. Ann Plast Surg 1986;17:503–512
37. Beyer CK, Fabian RL, Smith B. Naso-orbital fractures, complication and treatment. Ophthalmology 1982;89:456–463
38. Converse JM, Hogan VM. Open sky approach for reduction of naso-orbital fractures: case report. Plast Reconstr Surg 1970;46:396–398
39. Converse JM, Smith B. Naso-orbital fractures. Trans Am Acad Ophthalmol Otolaryngol 1976;80:622–623
40. Gross CW, Teague PF, Nakamura T. Reconstruction following severe nasofrontal injuries. Otolaryngol Clin North Am 1972;5:653–665
41. Becelli R, Renzi G, Mannino G, et al. Posttraumatic obstruction of lacrimal pathways: a retrospective analysis of 58 consecutive naso-orbitalethmoid fractures. J Craniofac Surg 2004;15:29–33
42. Gruss JS, Hurwitz JJ, Nik NA et al. The pattern and incidence of nasolacrimal injury in naso-orbital-ethmoid fractures: the role of delayed assessment and dacryocystorhinostomy. Br J Plast Surg 1985;38:116–121
43. Markowitz BL, Manson PN, Sargent LA et al. Management of the medial cantal tendon in nasoethmoid orbital fractures: the importance of the central fragment in classification and treatment. Plast Reconstr Surg 1991;87:843–853

44. Duvall AJ, Foster DA, Lyons DP et al. Medial canthoplasty: early and delayed repair. Laryngoscope 1981;91:173–183
45. Wulc AE, Arterberry JF. The pathogenesis of canalicular laceration. Ophthalmology 1991;98:1243–1249
46. Adenis JP. Management of canalicular trauma. Eye 1988; 2:223–225
47. Keith CG. Intubation of the lacrimal passages. Am J Ophthalmol 1968;70–74
48. Lauring L. Silicone intubation of the lacrimal system: pitfalls, problems and complications. Ann Ophthalmol 1976;8:489–498
49. MacGillivray RF, Stevens MR. Primary surgical repair of traumatic lacerations of the lacrimal canaliculi. Oral Surg Oral Med Oral Pathol 1996;81:157–163
50. Leone CR. Periorbital trauma. Int Ophthalmol Clin 1995;35:1–24
51. Hawes MJ, Segrest DR. Effectiveness of bicanalicular silicone intubation in the repair of canalicular lacerations. Ophthalmic Plast Surg 1985;1:185–190
52. Kersten RC, Kulwin DR. "One stitch" canalicular repair: a simplified approach for repair of canalicular laceration. Ophthalmology 1996;103:785–789
53. Reed S, Lissner G. Cinical study on the effectiveness of tear drainage with a single canalicular system under environmental stress. Ophthal Plast Reconstr Surg 1993;9:17–31
54. Welham RA. The immediate management of injuries to the lacrimal drainage apparatus. Trans Ophthalmol Soc UK 1982;102:216–217
55. Drnovsek-Olup B, Beltram M. Trauma of the lacrimal drainage system: retrospective study of 32 patients. Croatian Med J 2004;45:292–294
56. Ellis E III. Sequencing treatment of naso-orbitoethmoid fractures. J Oral Maxillofac Surg 1993;51:543–558
57. Stranc MF, Bunce AH. Dacryo-cystography in mid-facial fractures. Br J Plast Surg 1972;25:269–275
58. Unger JM. Fractures of the nasolacrimal fossa and canal: a CT study of appearance, associated injuries, and significance in 25 patients. AJR 1992;158:1321–1324
59. Glatt HJ. Evaluation of lacrimal obstruction secondary to facial fractures using computed tomography or computed tomographic dacryocystography. Ophthalmic Plast Reconstr Surg 1996;12:284–293
60. Ashenhurst M, Jaffer N, Hurwitz JJ et al. Combined computed tomography and dacryocystography for complex lacrimal problems. Can J Ophthalmol 1991;26:27–31

Chapter 10

Microsurgery of the Lacrimal System: Microendoscopic Techniques 10

Minimally Invasive Diagnostics and Therapy in Lacrimal Surgery

Karl-Heinz Emmerich, Ralf Ungerechts and Hans-Werner Meyer-Rüsenberg

Core Messages

- Transcanalicular endoscopy with ultrafine endoscopes has uncovered many new and previously unknown details in our understanding of lacrimal obstructions.
- In combination with different tools, such as the Erbium-YAG-laser and a special drill system in the simultaneous minimally invasive therapy of lacrimal obstructions, transcanalicular endoscopy represents a great advance in suitable cases and minimizes the rate of external DCR.

Contents

10.1 Introduction

It was not possible to view the lacrimal system directly until the 1990s. In all cases of stenosis of the lacrimal system the diagnosis depended on indirect procedures. Imaging procedures, such as dacryocystography with radio-opaque fluid, computer tomography, magnetic resonance tomography (MRT), high-resolution ultrasonography, and radionuclide-assisted procedures, have been of great importance in the operative therapy of lacrimal obstructions.

In cases of mechanical obstruction of the lacrimal system, surgical therapy is almost the only way to solve the problem of permanent epiphora.

The goal of lacrimal surgery without external scars led to the endonasal operation technique of internal dacryocystorhinostomy (DCR) according to West [6]. Over the years various modifications have been developed in this field, even in the past 20 years.The introduction of microscopes for endonasal surgery and flexible nasal endoscopes has considerably improved the results obtained. The combined approach of antegrade imaging and illumination of the lacrimal system with simultaneous endoscopically controlled endonasal preparation of the nasal mucosa, the bones, and the lacrimal sac has achieved excellent results. To minimize the operative trauma these endonasal techniques were supplemented with the use of various lasers such as holmium, KTP [Kaliumpotassium Titanylphosphate] or carbon dioxide [1, 2, 18, 21, 22].

To be able to select a suitable operative procedure in order to eliminate lacrimal obstruction, and to give an accurate prognosis, imaging is aimed at locating mechanical stenosis as precisely as possible. Operative trauma should be minimized and the benefits of the procedure can then be used optimally. The goal of being able to see pathological changes in the lacrimal passage directly led to the development of rigid and flexible endocanalicular endoscopes. The tight lumen of the canaliculi even in adults is scarcely more than 1 mm. This demands a high grade of miniaturization of the endoscopes; thus, the first endoscopes gave no satisfactory image quality and did not bring a true advance in diagnostics.

As a "spin-off" effect of the further developments in gastroduodenal endoscopes for endoscopic retrograde cholangiopancreatography (ERCP), superfine flexible endoscopes have reached a miniaturization of the diameter of down to 0.3 mm, which permits them to be used in transcanalicular diagnostics [10, 13]. The endoscopes with the smallest diameter of 0.3 mm had a possible transmission of 1500 pixels with the resulting pictures only of fair quality. By extending the diameter to 0.5 or 0.7 mm with a transmission of 3000 or 6000 pixels, a far better quality could be achieved. This was the beginning of a new phase in understanding the diseases of the lacrimal system. Direct assessment of changes of the mucosa was possible along with the detection of foreign bodies, dacryoliths, and tumors.

The next step was the development of miniaturized tools. Brought into the working channel as a probe, e.g., a laser fiber, a sling or a drill could be used. In this way new procedures to eliminate lacrimal obstructions have been developed, for example, laser dacryoplasty (LDP) and microdrill dacryoplasty (MDP) [9, 12, 14–17].

10.2 Dacryoendoscopy

10.2.1 Indication

Dacryoendoscopy should be performed before every kind of operation on the lacrimal system.

10.2.2 Contraindication

Children up to 1 year, and acute infections (e.g., dacryocystitis), are contraindications.

10.2.3 Instrumentation

10.2.3.1 Diagnostic Equipment

It was not possible to bring flexible endoscopes directly into the lacrimal system. The search to create a useful tool led to the modified Jünemann probe, developed from a Bangerter irrigation probe with a blunt tip and a diameter of 0.8 mm. This was developed to bring a channel into the lacrimal system for intubating the system with a silicone tube. The diameter of this probe was enlarged to 0.9 mm and a second channel for irrigation was added. The endoscope has a 70° angle view and a 0° direction view. The illumination is delivered by a high-power xenon cold light source connected to the camera by a TV adapter.

The camera has a residual light amplification and a high shutter speed of up to 1/2,000,000 s. The endoscopically generated picture is visible on a high-performance TV monitor (Fig. 10.1). During the endoscopic procedure the pictures can be recorded simultaneously through a video output and documented on an S-VHS video recorder or, more recently, a DVD/CD. The quality of the documentation is, however, reduced and the pictures in the text or presented by slides are of lesser quality. In spite of this, during the endoscopy the quality of the pictures is much improved.

Since the first lacrimal endoscopies, the system has had only minor changes, one change being the configuration of the endoscopes, e.g., the Vitroptic dacryoendoscope. The great advantage of this generation of endoscopes is that they do not need to be placed into the probe, for we have a fixed system; therefore, damage to the very sensitive and even expensive endoscopes can be avoided. Another step in the development of new endoscopes was the use of flexible probes as in the flexible Vitroptic dacryoendoscope (Figs. 10.2). Digitalization of the picture is improving the quality of the pictures up to now.

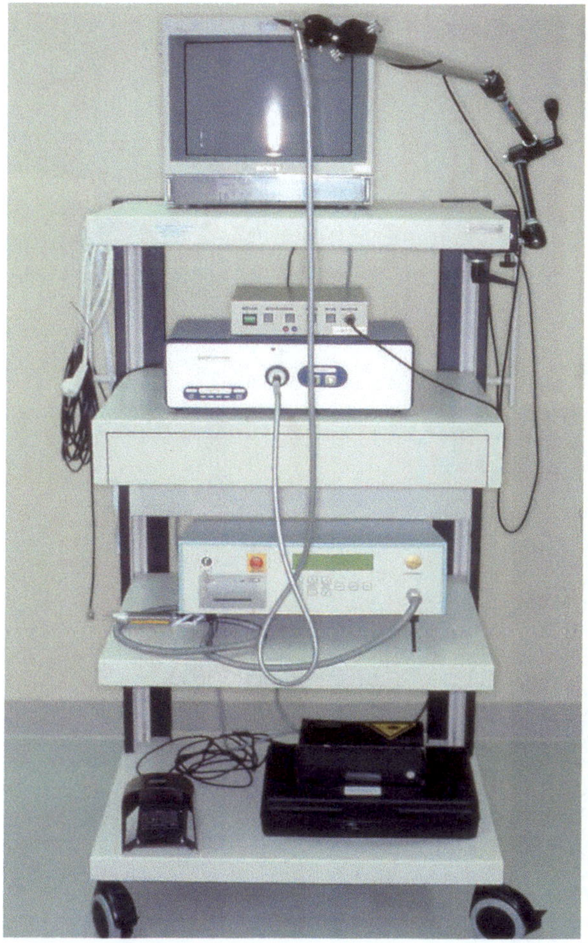

Fig. 10.1. Endoscopic system, featuring monitor, camera, xenon light source, Erbium-YAG laser, and video recorder

10.2.3.2 Therapeutic Equipment

First attempts at performing transcanalicular Laser-dacryoplasty (LDP) were carried out with a Holmium-YAG laser [11]. The laser probe was not connected to an endoscope. The diameter of the probe was 1.0 mm. With this laser probe a 1.0-mm cross section to the nose could be created in cases of canaliculus stenosis, but the results were not encouraging. The laser energy was 100 mJ and this energy was delivered by a quartz fiber.

To connect the fiber to the endoscope, the diameter of the fiber of the laser has to be very small (<0.4 mm); for example, this is possible with the semi-flexible fiber of a KTP laser [3]. The KTP laser is a solid-body crystal laser with an energy up to 10 W, which is very powerful. The released energy is sufficient for making bone holes, but the disadvantage is a certain thermal reaction with an enforced scarring reaction. This technique has shown the possibility of performing transcanalicular DCR, but because of this disadvantage it has been performed only in a small number of patients and has not established itself in other lacrimal centers.

Using a modified miniaturized Erbium-YAG laser developed for glaucoma surgery, a 375-mm sapphire fiber delivers the laser energy at the top of the probe up to a maximum of 50 mJ and a frequency of 1–3 Hz.

The length of the used laser fiber is 10–11 cm. The Erbium-YAG laser has a wavelength of 2.94 mm, a wavelength at which the maximum absorption is in water and the laser is operating photoablatively

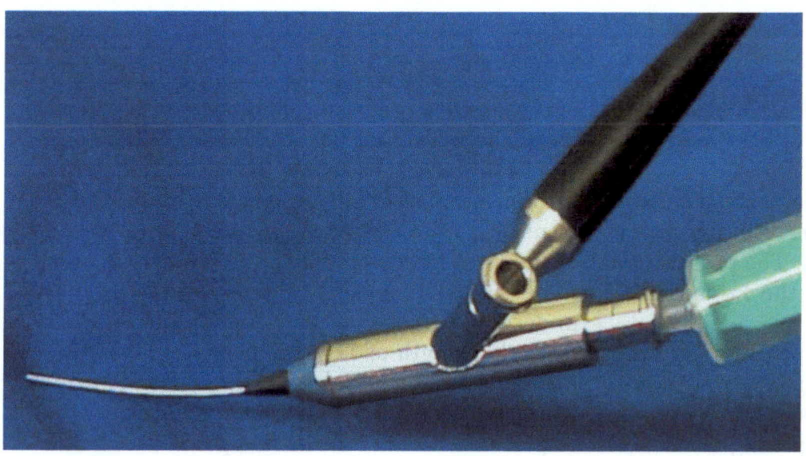

Fig. 10.2. Flexible endoscopic system "Titanflex" Vitroptic

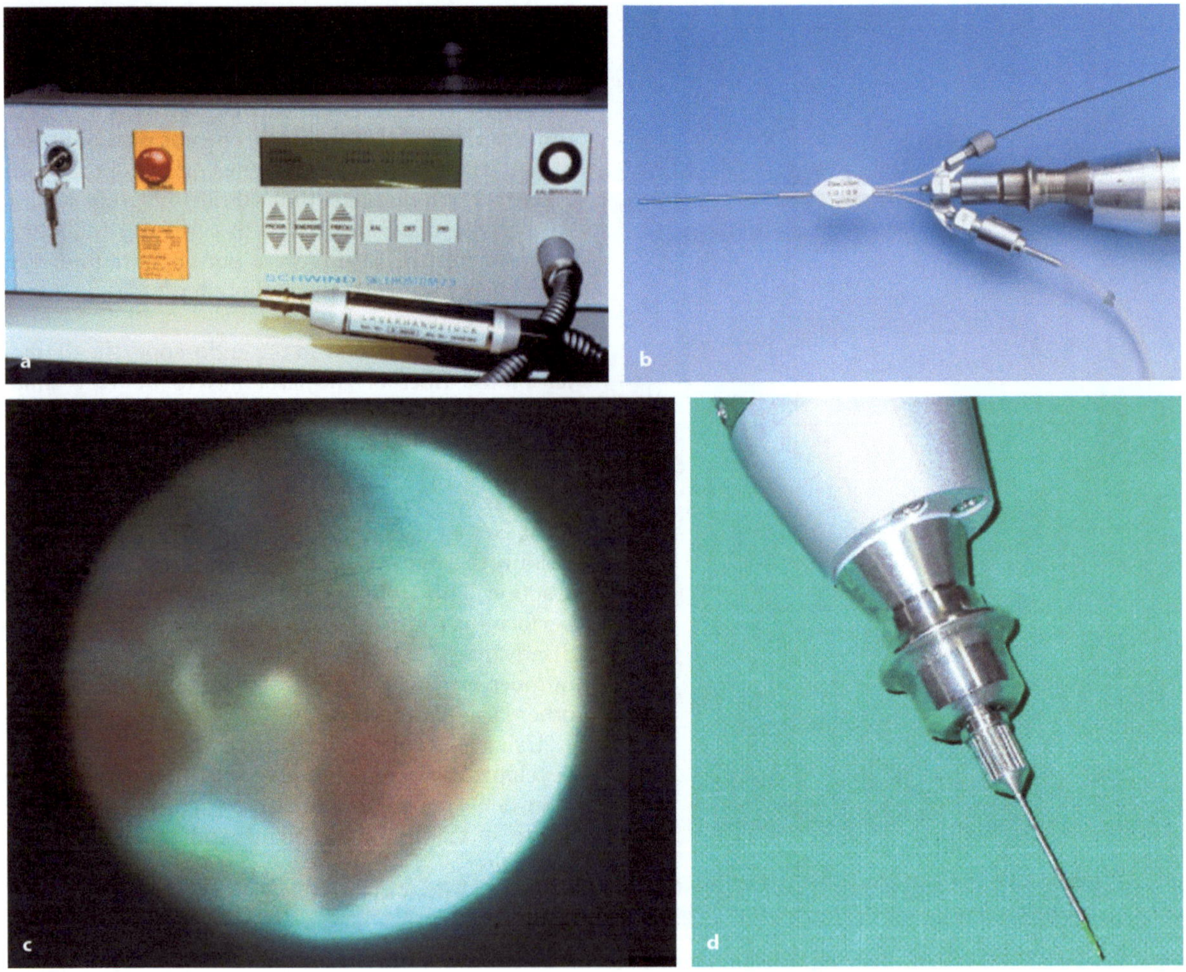

Fig. 10.3. a Erbium-YAG laser with miniaturized handpiece. b Three-channel probe, diameter 1.1 mm. c Endoscopic view of a laser probe in the lacrimal sac. d Sklerostom for treatment of canaliculus stenosis

(Fig. 10.3). The mucosal cells of the lacrimal sac have a water content of 80%, so the laser effect can be seen quickly.

The main effect of this laser in the lacrimal passage closed by the stenosis, however, is the resulting cavitation blister and not the ablation [4]. The preparation of bone holes is not possible with the Erbium-YAG laser.

The cavitation blister, which is caused by the laser impulse in the closed system, can extend over several millimeters. Punctal membranous stenosis can be opened by several impulses. The depth of penetration of the laser energy is only a few micrometers and the thermal effect is low.

The necrosis zone is only 10–20 μm and there is no carbonization. A modification of the Jünemann probe from two to three working channels allows placement of the laser fiber into the third channel and enables the laser treatment of the stenosis to be performed under endoscopic control. An additional short laser tip with a length of 4 cm has been used for the treatment of canalicular stenosis. This tip is not integrated in an endoscope. The endoscopic examination has to be performed before the laser application.

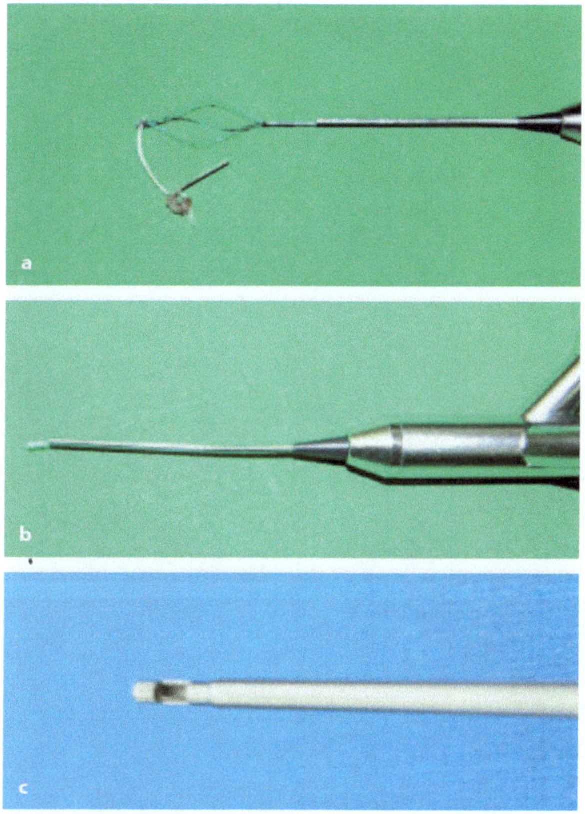

Fig. 10.4. Microendoscopic tools. a Sling for removal of foreign bodies. b Brush for taking cytological probes. c Plug for taking histological probes

Other microendoscopic tools have been already developed, such as a sling, to remove foreign bodies such as dacryoliths or remains of intubation material. There is even the possibility of taking biopsies with a plug or a brush (Fig. 10.4).

10.2.4 Anesthesia

It is possible to perform a dacryoendoscopy with anesthetizing eye drops by irrigating the lacrimal system with 4% cocaine solution and anesthetizing with a nasal spray. In our experience the endoscopy is best carried out before any surgical procedure, whether conventional or endoscopic. All these endoscopic procedures are performed with the patient under general anesthesia.

10.2.5 Operative Technique

In principle, performing an endoscopy in the lacrimal system is no more invasive than a deep probing of the lacrimal system. The puncta have to be dilated and it is useful to use an astringent solution some minutes before the endoscopy starts. Irrigating softly, the endoscope is inserted via the upper or lower canaliculus. The endoscope is pushed forward as far as possible as in normal lacrimal systems down to the inferior meatus, in other cases up to the point of stenosis. Unlike the endoscopies of the gastrointestinal system, the complete lacrimal passage can be judged by retracting the endoscope with simultaneous irrigation. Retracting and advancing the endoscope requires a certain amount of experience to obtain good pictures and to avoid a false passage. The learning curve is comparable to that for other endoscopic procedures such as gastroscopy, but even experienced examiners are not always able to get good pictures. In nearly every case, however, the additional information on the lacrimal system is useful.

In children under the age of 2 years the small diameter of the lacrimal system, especially of the punctum, increases the risk of injury; therefore, a purely diagnostic endoscopy should only be carried out in exceptional cases. Nevertheless, diseases of the lacrimal system in early childhood are mainly caused by malformations and in these cases the endoscopy cannot provide any essential additional information for the therapeutic procedure. Only in cases of failure following prior procedures should an endoscopy with subsequent endoscopic rechannelizing be performed to avoid a pediatric DCR [5].

10.2.5.1 Normal Findings

The endoscopic examination consists of observing various parts of the lacrimal system with different tissue formations such as the nasolacrimal duct, the lacrimal sac, and the canaliculi. In normal findings, the canalicular mucosa appears white and smooth. The canaliculi have a narrow lumen and a homogeneous structure of the walls (Fig. 10.5). The mucosa of the lacrimal sac is reddish, the lumen is wide, and the wall is structured by flat valves. During endoscopy, the production of mucus can soon be seen. After touching the mucosa, a small amount of bleeding on the surface can be noticed. If there is an inflamed sac,

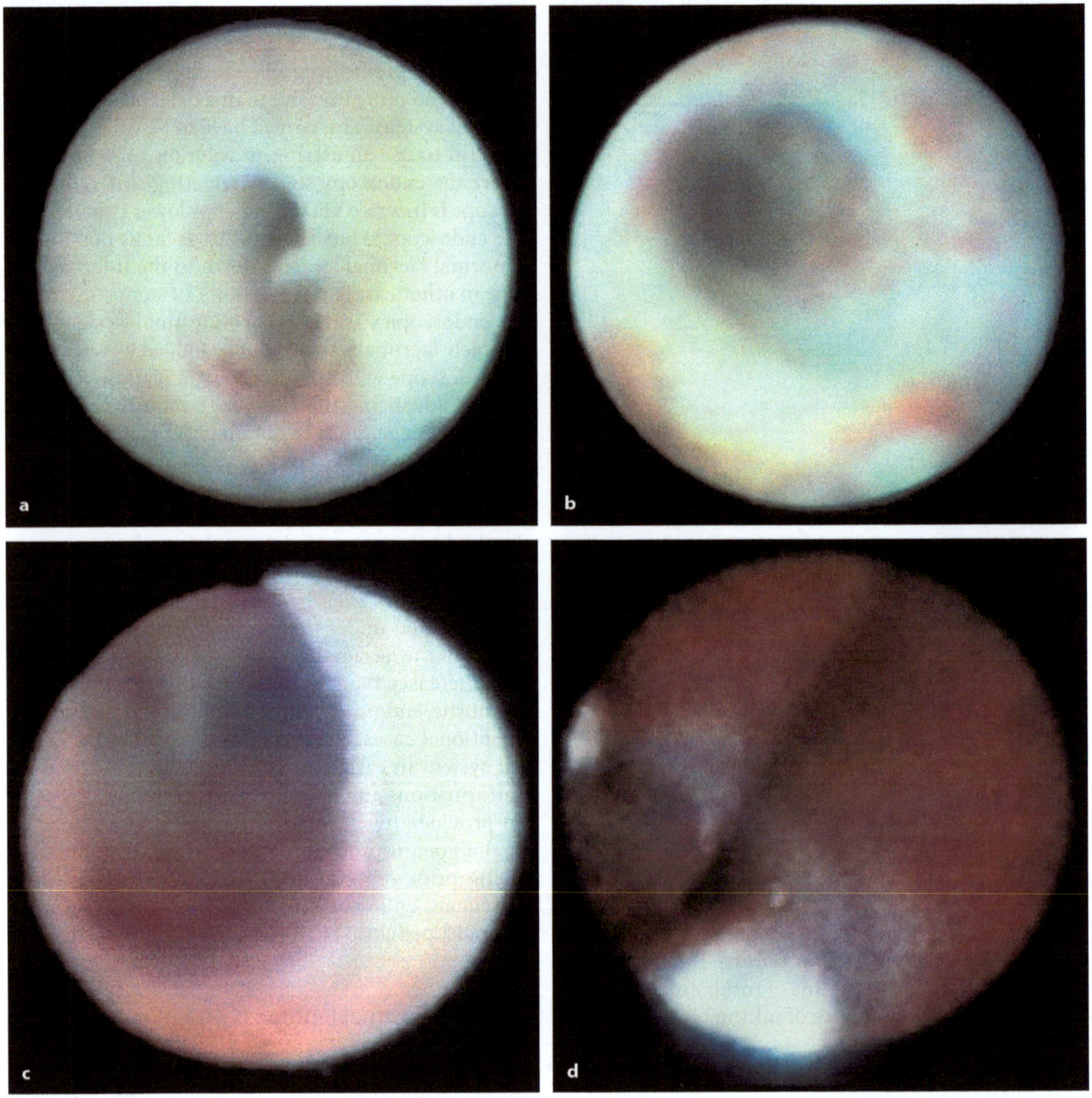

Fig. 10.5. Normal endoscopic findings of the lacrimal system. **a** Canaliculus. **b** Lacrimal sac. **c** Rosenmüller valve. **d** Nasal cavity

the bleeding is enforced. The transition from the canaliculi to the lacrimal sac shows the Rosenmüller valve.

This is a border between different histological structures of the canaliculi and the white squamous epithelium of the canaliculi and the transitional epithelium of the lacrimal sac. Between the lacrimal sac and the nasolacrimal duct, the Krause valve can be seen. The lumen in the nasolacrimal duct is narrow and shows no valves. The structure of the surface is reddish as in the lacrimal sac.

Polyps in the lacrimal sac can be identified. The nasal cavity is noticeable as an intensely red structure with a smooth surface and an enormous space [20].

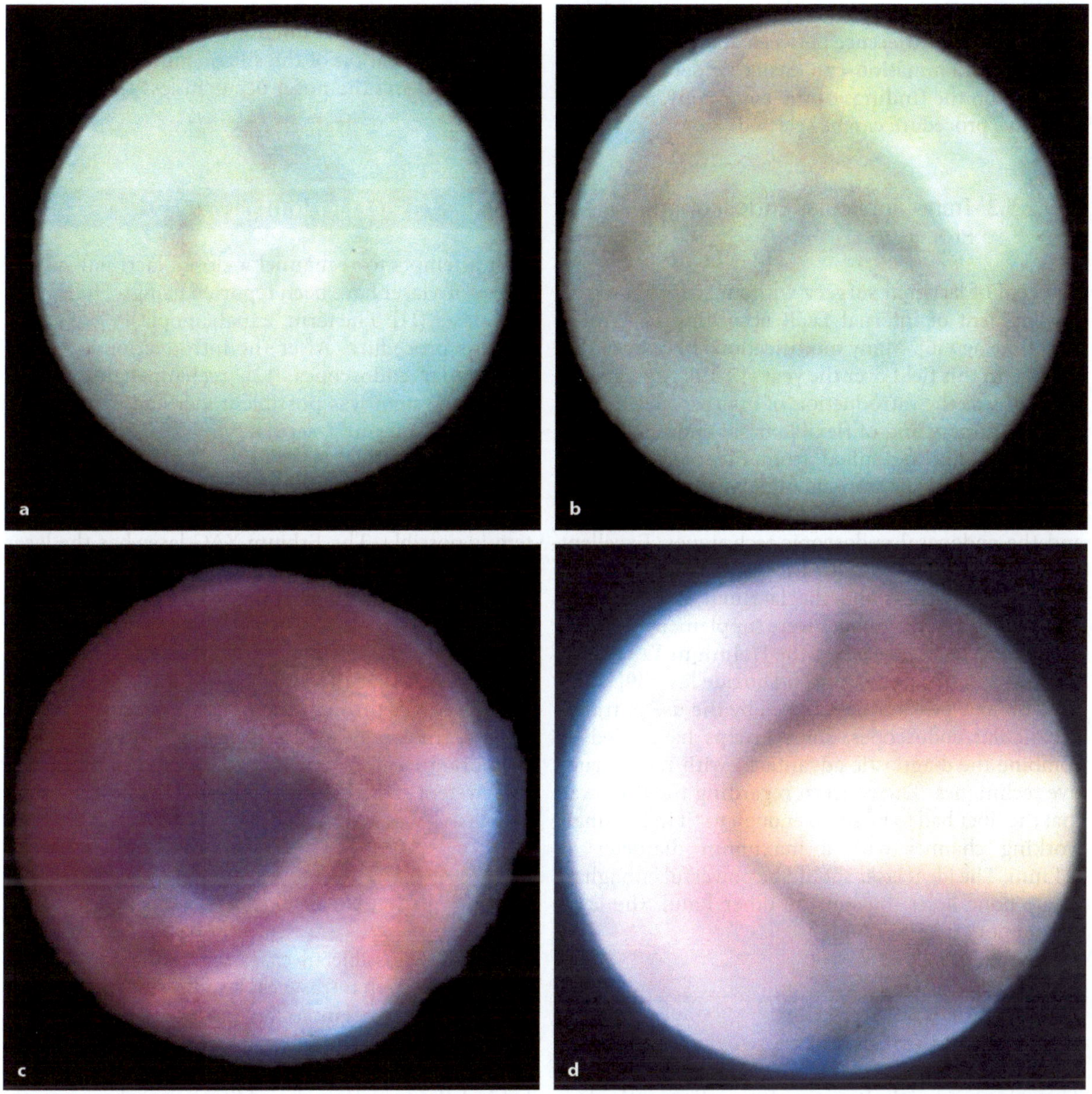

Fig. 10.6. Pathological findings. **a** Stenosis of the canaliculus. **b** Chronic dacryocystitis. **c** Acute dacryocystitis. **d** Rest of silicone tube after incomplete removal

10.2.5.2 Pathological Findings

Membranes surface scars, submucosal scar formations, and foreign bodies can be compared with normal findings (Fig. 10.6). Membranes can be seen in cases of chronic inflammations and are possible reasons for a subtotal closure of the lacrimal system, especially at the point of the pre-existing valves of Rosenmüller and Krause. A submucosal scar formation is characteristic of chronic inflammations with shrinking of the lacrimal sac. Polyps in the lacrimal sac can be identified. Remains of intubation material are a common reason for relapses and can easily be identified. The difference between acute and chronic mucosal inflammation can easily be seen, and depending on the findings of the endoscopy, a suitable operative procedure can be selected.

10.2.5.3 Transcanalicular Endoscopic Procedures

The goal of lacrimal surgery without scars led to the development of internal DCR according to West a long time ago [6]. Many modifications have been developed in this field over the years [7, 19]. A great step forward was the introduction of microscopes for endonasal surgery and of flexible nasal endoscopes [8]. New possibilities resulted from the combined approach of antegrade transcanalicular illumination by cold light sources developed for pars plana vitrectomy and the endonasal endoscopic techniques. Excellent results were achieved with the preparation of nasal mucosa, the bones, and the lacrimal sac. Some of these endonasal techniques were supplemented by the use of diverse lasers such as the Holmium-YAG laser, the KTP laser, and the Carbon Dioxide laser [9].

With new possibilities created by the use of transcanalicular endoscopes, some groups have tried to combine the diagnostic advantages with reconstructive techniques. The concern regarding the laser was that the fiber had to be small enough to fit in the small working channel with a maximum diameter of 0.4 mm. The ideal laser should be powerful enough to create bone holes, but on the other hand, the laser should not cause scarring.

10.2.6 Postoperative Care and Complications

There is no special aftercare after a diagnostic dacryoendoscopy.

Complications are as follows:

1. Recurrence of stenosis
2. Edema or hematoma of the eye lid because of a via falsa in approximately 2% of cases
3. Nose bleeding after removal of the silicone intubation in approximately 2% of cases
4. Slitting of the lacrimal punctum or spontaneous dislocation of the silicone intubation (e.g., by blowing the nose) occur in less than 5% of cases.

10.3 Laser Dacryoplasty

First attempts to rechannel a closed lacrimal system by use of a laser have been reported using a Holmium-YAG laser [11]. The term "canaliculoplasty" was used for this procedure. After the introduction of transcanalicular endoscopes [12], rechannelizing of the lacrimal system was possible under endoscopic control and the term "laser dacryoplasty" was used for this procedure [14, 15].

With regard to the diameter of the laser fiber, endoscopically controlled rechannelizing by a laser system is possible. The Erbium-YAG laser has the laser energy delivered by a sapphire fiber with a diameter of 375 mm. The glass fiber of a KTP laser is similar. In our experience we first started trying to perform a transcanalicular DCR with the Erbium-YAG laser but had to learn that the laser energy was not powerful enough to get through the bone to the nose. Nevertheless, the laser was useful enough to open closed membranes and in this way to open a blocked lacrimal system. For this procedure the term "laser dacryoplasty" was introduced.

10.3.1 Indications

An LDP is possible in cases of canalicular stenosis and high or deep intrasaccal lesions. The known anatomical valves seem to be the predilection points for adhesion of the valves, causing the closure in the lacrimal system typically 10–11 mm or 18–20 mm behind the punctum. In addition, membranous occlusions following a failed DCR can be treated successfully by LDP. Presently, LDP is mostly performed in cases of canalicular stenosis and in saccal stenosis. The mucosa of the lacrimal sac may not be acute inflamed with only a slightly enlarged diameter.

10.3.2 Contraindications

Laser dacryoplasty is not useful in cases of acute dacryocystitis, mucoceles, or widespread adhesions following viral infections such as herpes or lacrimal stenosis caused by bone displacement after midface fractures.

10.3.3 Erbium-YAG Laser Dacryoplasty

A modified miniaturized Erbium-YAG laser developed for glaucoma surgery has been in use since 1996 and delivers the laser energy by a sapphire fiber. In different parts the laser energy depends on the width of the laser fiber and with the used sapphire fiber of 375 mm an energy of 50 mJ with 1–3 Hz can be delivered at the top of the fiber. The absorption maximum of the Erbium-YAG laser is in water and the laser works photoablatively. The mucosal cells of the transitional epithelium of the lacrimal sac have a water content of nearly 80%, so the ablation results quickly. But there is not only the ablative effect: depending on the complete closure of the lacrimal system after the introduction of the endoscopic probe, a cavitation blister results of energy laser impulse and the edges of membranes and valves, which stick together, can be opened by the laser effect. The blister can extend over several millimeters and in this way punctal membranous stenosis can be opened with just a few pulses. In many cases this energy is powerful enough to open these membranous stenoses, but not too strong to make a false passage.

Initially, a diagnostic endoscopy is performed to check the indication for surgery. With complete stenosis of the lacrimal system without a mucocele there is an indication for LDP. The laser fiber is brought into an endoscope with a third working channel and the laser can be applied. After several laser impulses, free irrigation can be noted. Irrigation is now possible without the former resistance and the endoscopic picture confirms the opening. After opening the obstruction, bicanalicular intubation using a silicone tube with a diameter of 0.64 mm is carried out to prevent postoperative adhesions of the mucosa. The tubing remains in place usually for 3 months and is removed transcanalicularly (Fig. 10.7).

If there is no possibility of bicanalicular intubation, then a monocanalicular stent is used according to Fayet et al. [23]. This Monoka intubation remains in place for at least 6 weeks. The postoperative therapy is the same as that following bicanalicular intubation, which is performed easily in the clinical setting without general anesthesia.

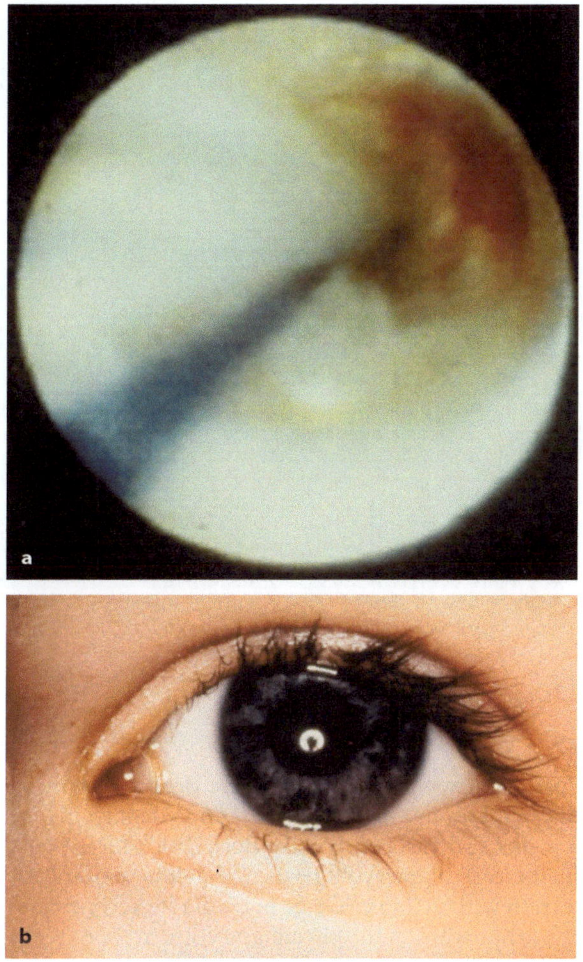

Fig. 10.7. **a** Laser dacryoplasty after intubation with silicone tube and Prolene file in the lacrimal sac. **b** Silicone intubation after LDP

Using this method, the success rate of LDP related to the indicating symptom epiphora is about 80% with a postoperative follow-up period of 20.4 months. As regards the canalicular stenosis only, the success rate is 67% and rises to 86% for isolated common canaliculus stenosis [16]. These LDP results in treatment of canalicular stenosis are better than those following other microsurgical procedures, even in the hands of experienced surgeons.

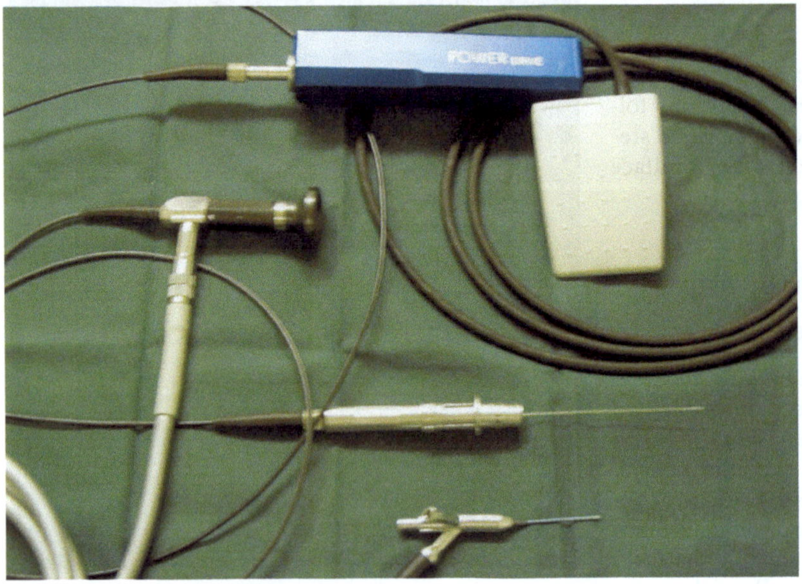

Fig. 10.8. Microdrill dacryoplasty system

10.3.4 Postoperative Care and Complications

Postoperatively we administer eye drops containing dexamethasone, polymyxin B, and neomycin for 3 weeks and vasoconstrictive nose drops for 1 week. In the case of dacryolithiasis and a concomitant infection with actinomyces or nocardia we recommend eye drops with erythromycin and colistin for 6 weeks and erythromycin orally for 10 days.

10.4 Microdrill Dacryoplasty

Immediately after the introduction of working transcanalicular dacryloplasty with the Erbium-YAG laser, Busse had the idea of introducing another tool into the third channel of the endoscope, namely a miniaturized drill (Fig. 10.8) [10, 17].

The concept was to construct a microdrill for transcanalicular manipulation under endoscopic view. The microdrill consisted of a stainless steel probe 0.3 mm in diameter which was driven by a battery-operated motor and a drill shaft. The frequency of the drill was 50 Hz. The drill was powered by a foot pedal and connected to a Vitroptic T, which is an endoscopic system where the endoscope has already been installed into the probe. In the meantime we have a much more powerful drill with a frequency up to 3000 Hz.

10.4.1 Indications

Indications for performing a microdrill dacryoplasty are removal of membranes or fragmentation and removal of dacryoliths. The microdrill dacryoplasty is particularly useful in the type of stenosis which has been first described by transcanalicular endoscopic findings as the "button-hole stenosis."

10.4.2 Contraindications

The contraindications are acute infections, mucocele, and stenosis after midfacial fractures.

10.4.3 MDP Procedure

The technique of microdrill dacryoplasty is similar to that of laser dacryoplasty. Initially, a diagnostic endoscopy is performed to check the indication. The drill is not powerful enough to create bone holes to perform a direct anastomosis between the lacrimal system and the nasal cavity; however, in many cases a

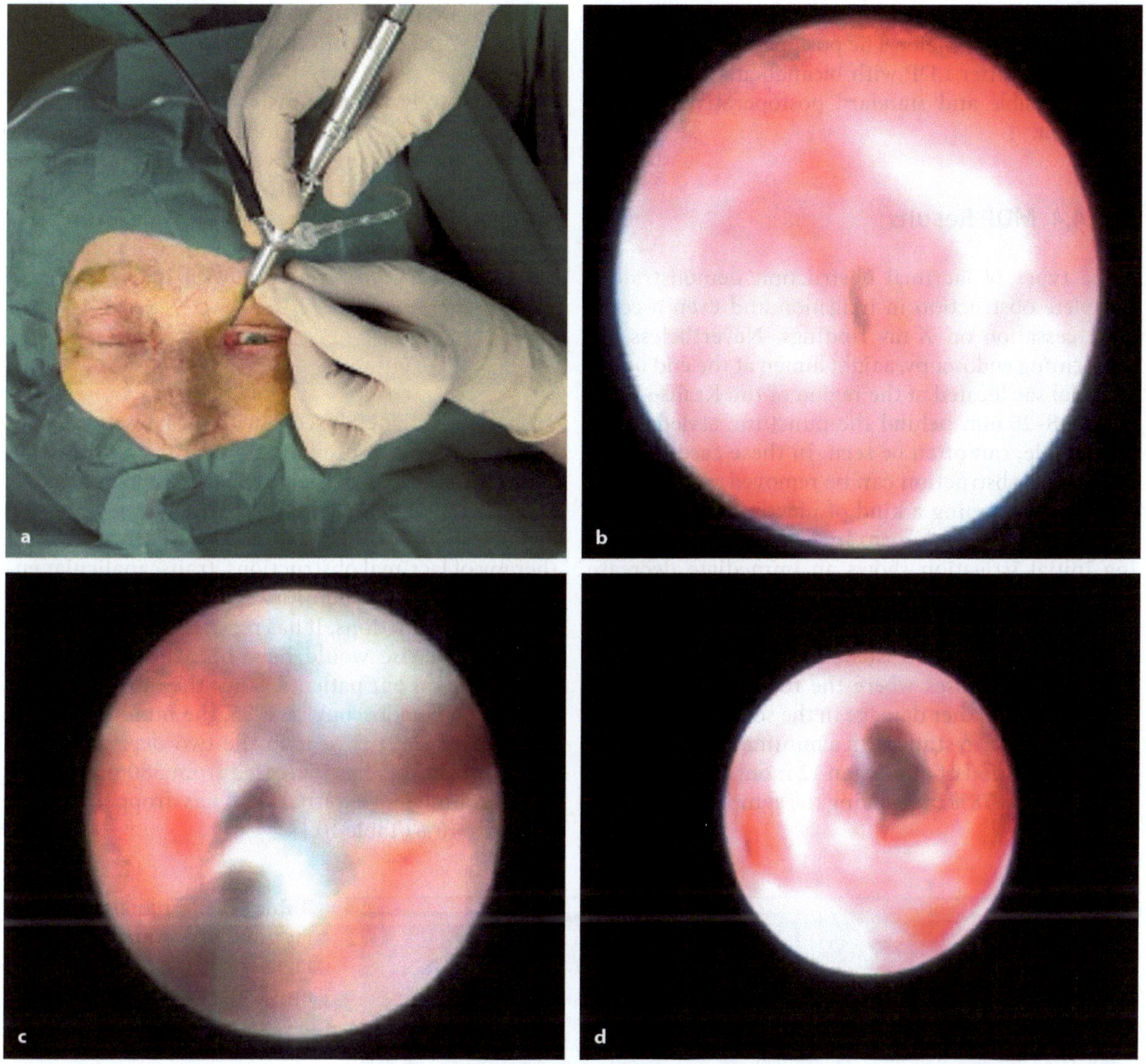

Fig. 10.9. a Performing microdrill dacryoplasty. b Subtotal stenosis at the end of the lacrimal sac. c Microdrill probe at work. d Subtotal stenosis after opening with microdrill

clinically completely closed system appears endoscopically not to be completely closed and shows a buttonhole-like closure with a partial lumen. In such cases a complete opening of the system is possible and can be performed by microdrill dacryoplasty (MDP).

The first step in performing a MDP is dilation of the upper or lower punctum in order to insert the Vitroptic T into the lacrimal system (Fig. 10.9). The diameter of the system is 1.1 mm, so that the procedure is possible even in children 2 years or older. Under endoscopic control, the microdrill is brought up to the location of the stenosis and pulled forward in front of the optic.

A continuous irrigation is required in order to prevent lacerations and to control the success of the procedure. After removing all the obstructions, success is again assessed by irrigation under endoscopic control.

It is possible to compare the irrigation resistance by a special manometer. The postoperative regimen is the same as after LDP with bicanalicular intubation when possible and standard postoperative medical treatment.

10.4.4 MDP Results

Some types of lacrimal obstruction demonstrate a complete obstruction in irrigation and even a complete cessation on X-ray findings. Nevertheless, by performing endoscopy, a tight lumen at the end of the lacrimal sac located at the region of the Krause valve about 18–20 mm behind the punctum, styled like a buttonhole, can often be seen. In these cases in particular the obstruction can be removed with the microdrill performing a kind of mucosa curettage and enlarging the tight lumen. Increased resistance during initial irrigation shows an immediate decrease after a successful microdrill application. According to this model, the microdrill is not suitable for the treatment of complete stenoses, and especially for canalicular stenoses where the rotation of the drill might cause further damage in the soft tissues.

In a long-term study with a minimal postoperative follow-up period of more than 12 months, the success rate is almost 78% in reducing the symptom of epiphora.

10.4.5 Postoperative Care and Complications

Postoperatively we administer eye drops containing dexamethasone, polymyxin B, and neomycin for 3 weeks, and vasoconstrictive nose drops for 1 week.

In the case of dacryolithiasis and a concomitant infection with actinomyces or nocardia we recommend eye drops with erythromycin and colistin for 6 weeks and erythromycin orally for 10 days.

10.5 Conclusion

Transcanalicular endoscopy with the new endoscopes has been useful in providing much new information about the anatomy of the lacrimal drainage pathways and the causes of lacrimal obstructions. Combining different tools for the simultaneous minimal invasive therapy of lacrimal obstructions, transcanalicular endoscopy is a great step forward in the treatment of lacrimal obstructions. It has reduced the rate of DCR, which otherwise would have been necessary to be performed on our patients. Since the introduction of the lacrimal endoscopy in 1995, the number of lacrimal procedures per year in the two departments of the main authors has increased from 380 up to 1600, but the number of external DCR has dropped from 30 to nearly 10% (Table 10.1).

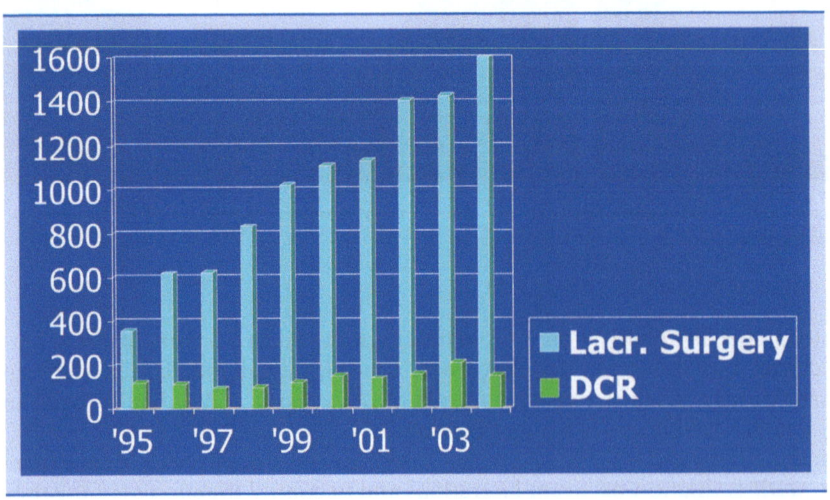

Table 10.1. Frequency of lacrimal procedures in the lacrimal centers of Hagen and Darmstadt (Germany)

Even if the success rate after laser dacryoplasty and MDP is no higher than 80%, this rate is very reasonable for a minimally invasive first-step procedure with a low rate of possible complications.

Lacrimal endoscopy has provided new insights into the pathology of the diseases of obstruction and the morphology of the lacrimal system. With endoscopy we can see and decide at once what to do and are able to perform minimally invasive therapy with the best results for the patient. In the past only clinical impression indirect imaging gave suggestions as to what was possible, and in many cases the surgeon was surprised but not amused during surgery. Minimally invasive therapy with laser or drill is a great advance in the management of the problems of lacrimal disorders.

Reference

1. Bartley GB (1994) The pros and cons of laser dacrycysto rhinostomy. Am J Ophthalmol 117:103–106
2. Emmerich KH, Busse H, Meyer-Rüsenberg HW, Hörstensmeyer CG (1997) External dacryocystorhinostomy: indications, method, complications and results. Orbit 16:25–29
3. Müllner K, Wolf G, Luxenberg W, Hofmann T (2001) Laser assistierte transkanalikuläre Dakryozystorhinostomie. Ophthalmologe 98:174–177
4. Mrochen M, Riedel P, Donitzky C, Seiler T (2001) Zur Entstehung von Kavitationsblasen bei der Erbium-YAG-Laser-Vitrektomie. Ophthalmologe 98:163–167
5. Emmerich KH, Meyer-Rüsenberg HW (2002) Erkrankungen der ableitenden Tränenwege im Kindesalter. Z prakt. Augenheilkunde 23:19–27
6. West JM (1914) A window resection of the nasal duct in cases of stenosis. Trans Am Ophthalmol Soc 12:654
7. Berryhill BH (1982) Twenty years experience with intranasal transseptal dacryocystorhinostomy. Laryngoscopy 92:379–381
8. Lindberg JV, Anderson RL, Bumsted RM, Barreres R (1982) Study of intranasal ostium external dacryocystorhinostomy. Arch Ophthalmol 100:1758–1762
9. Gonnering RS, Lyon DB, Fisher JC (1991) Endoscopic laser-assisted lacrimal surgery. Am J Ophthalmol 111:152–157
10. Emmerich KH, Meyer-Rüsenberg HW (2001) Endoskopische Tränenwegschirurgie. Ophthalmologe 98:607–612
11. Dutton JJ, Holck DE (1996) Holmium laser canaliculoplasty. Ophthal Plast Reconstr Surg 12: 211–217
12. Kuchar A, Novak P, Pieh S, Fink M, Steinkogler FJ (1999) Endoscopic laser recanalisation of presaccal canalicular obstruction. Br J Ophthalmol 83:443–447
13. Kuchar A, Novak P, Ofuoglu A, Steinkogler FJ (1995) Die Endoskopie der ableitenden Tränenwege. Spektrum Augenheilkunde 9:187–189
14. Emmerich KH, Lüchtenberg M, Meyer-Rüsenberg HW, Steinhauer J (1997) Dakryoendoskopie and Laserdakryoplastik: Technik und Ergebnisse. Klin Monatsbl Augenheilkunde 211:375–379
15. Meyer-Rüsenberg HW, Emmerich KH, Lüchtenberg M, Steinhauer J (1999) Endoskopische Laserdakryoplastik. Methodik und Ergebnisse nach drei Monaten. Ophthalmologe 96:332–334
16. Steinhauer J, Norda A, Emmerich KH, Meyer-Rüsenberg HW (2000) Laserkanalikuloplastik. Ophthalmologe 97:692–695
17. Emmerich KH, Ungerechts R, Meyer-Rüsenberg HW (2000) Possibilities and limits of minimal invasive lacrimal surgery. Orbit 19:67–71
18. Caldwell GW (1893) A new operation for the radical cure of obstruction of the nasal duct. N Y Med J 58:476
19. Busse H, Hollwich F (1977) Kurz- und Langzeitergebnisse dacryocystorhinostomia externa nach Kaleff-Hollwich. Klin Monatsbl Augenheilkd 171:986–989
20. Jünemann G, Schulte D (1975) Ursachen und Therapie der Stenosen der abführenden Tränenwege des Erwachsenen. In: Meyer-Schwickerath G, Ullrich (eds) Moderne Probleme der Erkrankungen der Lider und des Tränenapparates, 1st edn. Enke, Stuttgart, pp 243–264
21. Massaro BM, Gonnering RS, Harris GJ (1990) Endonasal laser dacryocystorhinostomy. A new approach to nasolacrimal obstruction. Arch Ophthalmol 108:1172–1176
22. Welham RA, Wulc AE (1987) Management of unsuccessful lacrimal surgery. Br J Ophthalmol 71:152–157
23. Fayet B, Assouline M, Bernard JA (1998) Monocanalicular nasolacrimal duct intubation. Ophthalmology 105:1795–1796

Chapter 11

Conjunctivorhinostomy

Werner J. Heppt

11

Core Messages

- Conjunctivorhinostomy is indicated in patients suffering from an obliteration of the upper and lower lacrimal duct creating a lacrimal bypass between the fornix of the conjunctiva and the nasal cavity.
- The use of pedicled mucosal-lined tract techniques with temporary stenting are superior to free grafting providing primary healing with less granuloma tissue and cicatricial formation and a reduced degree of osseous proliferation in the area of the osteal perforation.
- The combination of a conjunctival flap with a cartilage-containing nasal septal flap acting as a permanent autogenous stent of the new passage seems to be the most effective surgical way.

Contents

11.1 Introduction

In the treatment of lacrimal duct stenosis the main parameters to be focused on are cause, localization, and prior treatment of the obstruction. Endonasal dacryocystorhinostomy is the most common procedure in lacrimal drainage surgery indicated in obliterations of the lower lacrimal tract (Weidenbecher et al. 1994; Sham and van Hasselt 2000). For the repair of the upper lacrimal apparatus a variety of delicate procedures have been published. Partial integrity of the canaliculi and/or the adjacent lacrimal sac provided silicone intubation (Patel 2000), canaliculodacryocystorhinostomy (Doucet and Hurwitz 1982), fundal transposition, or conjunctivodacryocystorhinostomy including synthetic tubing (Jones 1965; Glatt and Puttermann 2000) have to be taken into consideration. Complete absence of functional upper and lower lacrimal duct structures requires a total lacrimal bypass from the conjunctival sac to the nasal cavity. Even the connection from the conjunctiva to the mediosuperior corner of the antrum may be feasible in special cases (Huang et al. 1992); however, considering physiology of the medially oriented tear flow, conjunctivorhinostomy is the method of choice for the creation of a complete lacrimal bypass (Marube del Castillo 1982; Nissen and Sorensen 1987; Walter 1997).

Within the past decades many techniques have been developed for reconstruction of the mucosal lining of the new passage, which is the key of the procedure. Attempts with free grafting of vein (Soll 1983) or buccal mucosa (Campell 1983) failed due to secondary intention healing, granuloma tissue formation, and cicatrical changes resulting in restenosis in a high percentage. Facing these problems Welham (1987) and Arden et al. (1990) described nasal and conjunctival flaps with the advantages of primary healing and temporary stenting. In 2003 a case report was published by Yung and Hardman-Lea (2003) describing a pedicle nasal septal tube for the reconstruction of lacrimal drainage passage.

In the following a survey is given on the most common techniques of conjunctivorhinostomy concentrating on the combination of a conjunctival flap and a cartilage containing nasal septal flap (Walter 1997).

11.2 Indications

11

The conjunctivorhinostomy is indicated in patients suffering from epiphora and chronic conjunctival irritation caused by an obliteration of the upper lacrimal tract and a complete non-functional lower passage. It is also indicated when a conjunctivodacryocystorhinostomy failed in repairing a canalicular stenosis with intact lower lacrimal system or when a restenosis occurs after previous dacryocystorhinostomy in patients with saccal and postsaccal stenosis. This may be true for patients who underwent severe trauma of the eyelids and/or of the naso-orbital bony complex. Furthermore, complete obliterations may occur in chronic inflammations, congenital abnormalities, irradiations, and in defects owing to the resection of malignant tumors. Finally, many patients with lacrimal duct obliteration belong to the idiopathic group with no detectable reason.

11.3 Contraindications

In patients with saccal and postsaccal stenosis, other, less invasive procedures (see other chapters of the book) are primarily indicated.

11.4 Operative Techniques

11.4.1 Basic Procedure

The conjunctivorhinostomy is one of the most challenging techniques in lacrimal duct repair creating a lacrimal passage between the fornix of the conjunctiva and the nasal cavity. Requiring delicate and tedious dissection, the procedure should be performed under general anesthesia. After application of vasoconstrictors to the nasal mucosa and local infiltration of the lateral nasal wall using 1% xylocain with 1:100,000 epinephrine, the skin of the medial canthal area is incised in a curvilinear fashion from the level of the medial canthal ligament along to the orbital rim (Fig. 11.1 a). This is followed by cauterization of the angular vessels and by incision and elevation of the periosteum of the lateral nasal wall, the medial orbital wall, and the frontal process of the maxilla. The ex-

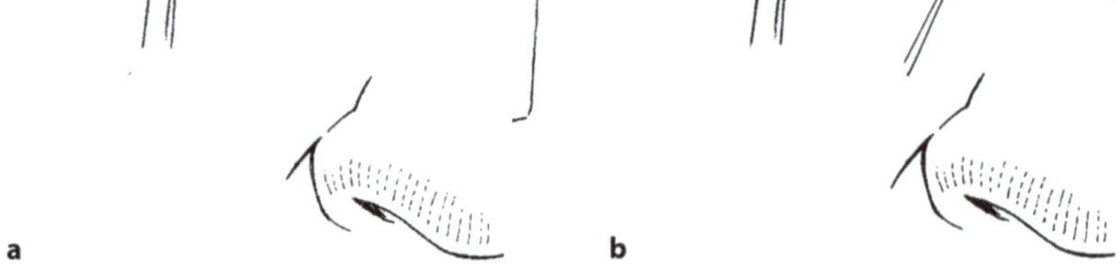

Fig. 11.1. Basic procedures in conjunctivorhinostomy. **a** Curvilinear skin incision from the area of the medial canthal ligament along the orbital rim. **b** External rhinostomy: removal of the exposed bone below the medial canthal ligament and along the orbital rim using a diamond drill

posed bone below the medial canthal ligament, along the orbital rim is removed in an area of about 1.5 cm in diameter using a diamond drill (Fig. 11 b). Taking off the bone special attention has to be paid in the preservation of the underlying nasal mucosa. For better exposure of the nasal mucosa the middle turbinate should be fractured medially from an endonasal approach. Once the osteal perforation has been completed an incision of the infero-medial fornix of the conjunctiva is done in a line just below the caruncle along the orbital rim. This is followed by blunt dissection behind the orbital septum and underneath the lacrimal sac creating a tunnel to the osseous perforation.

For the creation of the mucosal lining of the new lacrimal passage there are three options.

11.4.2 Bipedicled Nasal Mucosal Flap

According to the dacryo-fornix-rhinostomy described by Murube del Castillo (1992) a cranially pedicled nasal mucosal flap extending from the orbital rim to the nasal valve area is fashioned (Fig. 11.2 a); therefore, the nasal mucosa inferior, medial, and lateral to the osseous perforation is detached from the overlying bone using an blunt spatula with a curved end. The flap is externalized through the osseous window and divided into two parts: a superiorly based superomedial flap for reconstruction of the posterior wall of the passage and a laterally based inferolateral flap for reconstruction of the anterior wall (Fig. 11.2 a). The flaps are sutured to the corresponding posterior and anterior lip of the conjunctival incision and stented with a semirigid silicon sheet 1.5 cm wide and 5 cm long (Fig. 11.2 b, c). The stent may be removed a few days after surgery.

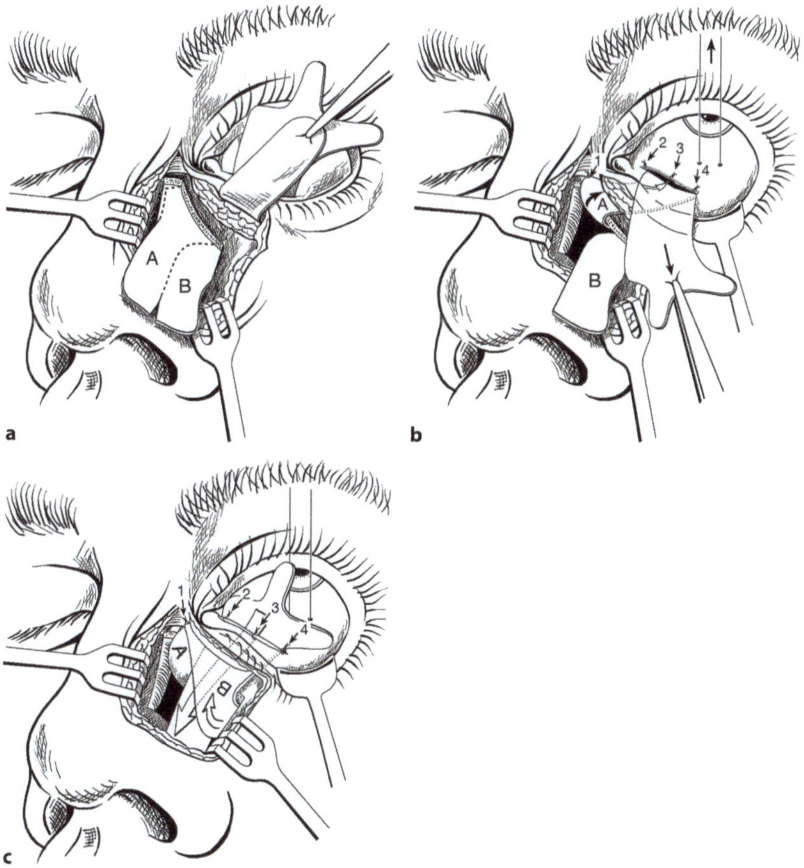

Fig. 11.2. Bipedicled nasal mucosal flap. a Division of the externalized nasal mucosa in a superiorly based superomedial flap (*A*) and a laterally based inferolateral flap (*B*). A silicon band is passed through the wound, and its two ends are fixed with a forceps. b The superomedial flap is reverted and sutured to the inferior edge of the tendo-oculi (*1*) and the posterior lip of the conjunctival wound (*2–4*), with its epithelial surface forward. c The inferolateral flap (*B*) is rotated, maintaining its epithelial face backwards. Its distal end is sutured to the inferior edge of the tendo-oculi (*1*) and to the anterior lip of the conjunctival wound (*2–4*). (From Murube 1992)

11.4.3 Conjunctival and Nasal Flap With Stenting

After osseous perforation, incision of the conjunctiva, and creation of a connecting subcutaneous tunnel, an U-shaped incision is done to fashion a posterolaterally based nasal mucosal flap of about 1×2-cm dimension (Fig. 11.3 a; Arden 1990). The flap is rotated upward to reconstruct the superoposterior wall of the new conduit. For complete mucosal lining of the new conduit a medially based flap is elevated from the medial conjunctiva. It is rotated downward repairing the anteroinferior side of the wall (Fig. 11.3 a; Arden 1990). Alternatively, the flap may be raised from the lower palpebral conjunctiva, 5 mm in the anteroposterior dimension and 15 mm in horizontal length (Huang 1992). Both flaps are sutured around a silicone tube of at least 2 mm in diameter facing the mucosal layer inward (Fig. 11.3 b). For approximation of the mucosal edges 5-0 absorbable sutures are recommended. After correct positioning of the tube under endonasal endoscopic control, the skin is closed in layers. Depending on the healing process, the tube will be removed between weeks 3 and 6. Only in certain cases of restenosis or severe scarring may it be indicated to leave the tube for a longer period. Nevertheless, without proper handling, tube dislodgement, infection, granuloma tissue, and scar formations may result from alloplastic material.

11

11.4.4 Conjunctival and Cartilage Containing Nasal Septal Flap

This technique provides a complete mucosal lining of the new conduit with additional cartilaginous support (Walter 1997). For reconstruction of the anterosuperior wall a conjunctival flap is harvested from the lower palpebral conjunctiva (Fig. 11.4 a). Dimensions of the rectangular, medially based flap are about 15 mm in horizontal length and 5 mm in width. After dissection of a subcutaneous tunnel the flap is rotated downward to the osseus perforation (Fig. 11.4 b). Reconstruction of the inferoposterior wall is done by a cranially pedicled mucoperichondrial nasal septal flap. The flap is fashioned via an endonasal approach containing cartilage of the anterior part of the nasal septum at its distal end (Fig. 11.4 b). Harvesting the cartilage, the perichondrium and mucosa of the opposite septum have to be preserved meticulously. After thinning of the cartilage using a 15 blade, the flap (1 cm in width and 3–4 cm in length) is rotated upward and sutured to the posterior margin of the incised conjunctiva using 5-0 absorbable threads (Fig. 11.4 c); thus, the cartilage lies in the critical area of the osteal perforation supporting the inferoposterior wall of the new lacrimal passage. Finally, the lateral margins of both flaps are approximated and the conjunctival flap is sutured to an inferiorly based flap of the lateral nasal wall. For short stenting of the new passage a soft silicone tube is inserted for about 10 days (Fig. 11.4 d).

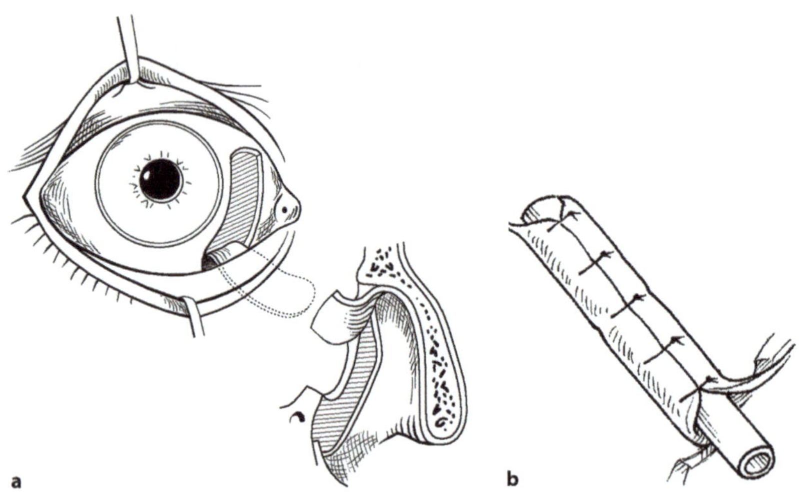

Fig. 11.3. Medial bulbar conjunctival and nasal mucosal flap. **a** Design of both flaps. **b** Tubulization of the conjunctival and nasal mucosal flap about Jones tube after rotation and end-to-end anastomoses. (From Arden 1990)

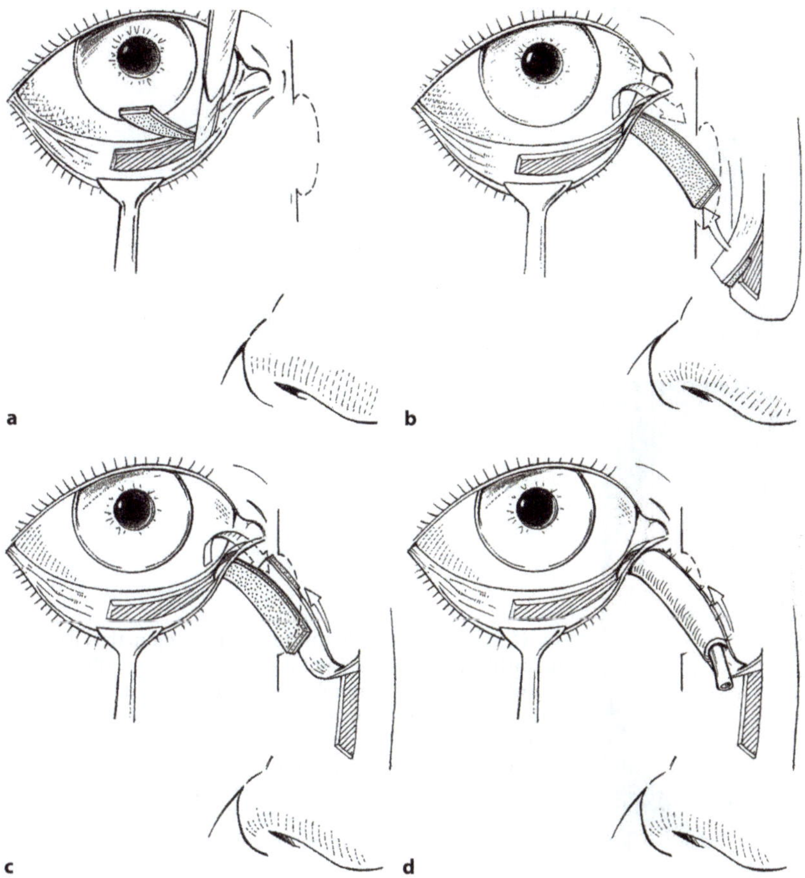

Fig. 11.4. Conjunctival flap and cartilage containing nasal septal flap. **a** A conjunctival flap is harvested from the lower palpebral conjunctiva. **b** Rotation of the conjunctival flap downward to the osseous perforation and elevation of a cartilage containing nasal septal flap. **c** Upward rotation of the nasal septal flap. Suturing of the cartilage containing distal end to the posterior lip of the conjunctival incision. **d** Temporary stenting of the new lacrimal bypass. (From Walter 1997)

The donor defect in the lower palpebral conjunctiva is closed using inverted fashioned 6-0 absorbable sutures, whereas the donor site in the nasal septum may be left for secondary intention healing. To control bleeding a nasal package is recommended for 1 day.

11.5 Postoperative Care and Complications

Prophylactic antibiotics are administered for the first week after surgery. Usually 3 months postoperatively, after complete epithelialization of the new lacrimal bypass nasal septal flaps' pedicle may be severed.

Drawbacks of tube stenting may be dislodgement, extrusion, granulation tissue formation, adhesions, nasal, and conjunctival irritation; therefore, stenting of the new duct should be avoided and practiced only for a short time when needed.

Careful and sufficient dissection ensures that all described techniques are at lower risk for corneal or scleral injuries as well as for secondary limitations of eye movements.

Although conjunctivorhinostomy with flaps of the lateral nasal wall and/or the conjunctiva with additional temporary stenting are commonly considered to be most effective in managing severe tear-duct dysfunction, they may be associated with secondary-intention healing and severe scarring. The most critical area for the development of a restenosis is the posterior wall of the new conduit next to the osseus perforation and the anterior ethmoid. Support of the lacrimal bypass by a cartilage-containing nasal septal flap provides autologous stenting of this area. Consequently, the risk for restenosis may be reduced.

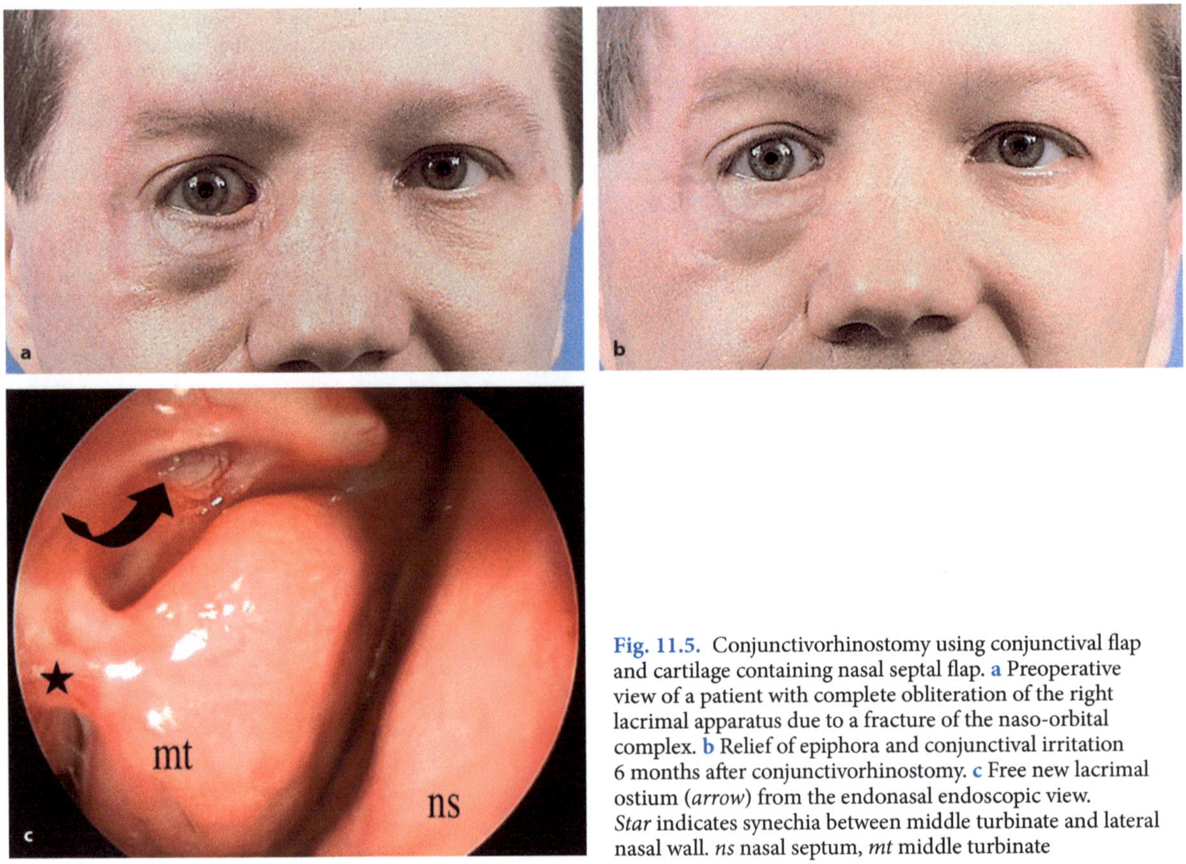

Fig. 11.5. Conjunctivorhinostomy using conjunctival flap and cartilage containing nasal septal flap. **a** Preoperative view of a patient with complete obliteration of the right lacrimal apparatus due to a fracture of the naso-orbital complex. **b** Relief of epiphora and conjunctival irritation 6 months after conjunctivorhinostomy. **c** Free new lacrimal ostium (*arrow*) from the endonasal endoscopic view. *Star* indicates synechia between middle turbinate and lateral nasal wall. *ns* nasal septum, *mt* middle turbinate

11.6 Outcome

The use of pedicled mucosal-lined tract techniques enables primary healing with less granuloma tissue and cicatricial formation and a minor degree of osseus proliferation in the area of the osteal perforation. Compared with free grafting of buccal mucosa or vein, the pedicle of the flaps puts graft take at lower risk. Preservation of the medial canthal ligament and of the caruncle prevents asymmetry. Due to its capillary attraction and the action of gravity, the medio-vertical-oriented passage provides tear drainage under physiology-like conditions. Movements of the eyeball and blinking result in changes of the pressure in the fornix supporting the pump mechanics of the eye.

Clinical findings and the endoscopic assessment of the fluorescein flow into the nasal cavity show the technique to be highly efficient with relief of epiphora and conjunctival irritation in a high percentage (Fig. 11.5a–c). Nevertheless, there is a lack of valid statistical data proving the efficacy of tear drainage quantitatively, which is true even for other techniques in conjunctivorhinostomy.

11.7 Highlights

The conjunctivorhinostomy is indicated in patients suffering from an obliteration of the upper and lower lacrimal duct creating a lacrimal bypass between the fornix of the conjunctiva and the nasal cavity. Furthermore, it has been found to be a reliable treatment option when a conjunctivodacryocystorhinostomy failed in repairing a canalicular stenosis with intact lower lacrimal system or when a restenosis occurs after previous dacryocystorhinostomy in patients with saccal and postsaccal stenosis.

Considering the various complications in the reconstruction of the new lacrimal duct, the use of pedicled mucosal-lined tract techniques with temporary stenting is superior to free grafting, providing primary healing with less granuloma tissue and cicatricial formation and a reduced degree of osseus proliferation in the area of the osteal perforation. In the present authors' opinion, among all surgical techniques the combination of a conjunctival flap with a cartilage-containing nasal septal flap acting as a permanent autogenous stent of the new passage seems to be the most effective surgical method.

Reference

Arden RL, Mathog RH, Nesi FA (1990) Flap reconstruction techniques in conjunctivorhinostomy. Otolaryngol Head Neck Surg 102:150–155

Campell CB, Shannon GM, Flanagan JC (1983) Conjunctivodacryocystorhinostomy with mucous membrane graft. Ophthalmic Surg 14:647–652

Doucet TW, Hurwitz JJ (1982) Canaliculodacryocystorhinostomy in the management of unsuccessful lacrimal surgery. Arch Ophthalmol 100:619–621

Glatt HJ, Puttermann AM (2000) Conjunctivodacryocystorhinostomy. In: Mauriello JA Jr (ed) Unfavorable results of eyelid and lacrimal surgery. Butterworth-Heinemann, Oxford, pp 575–589

Huang TT, Sasaki K, Nozaki M (1992) Reconstruction of the lacrimal excretory system. Plast Reconstr Surg 90:399–404

Jones LT (1965) Conjunctivodacryocystorhinostomy. Am J Ophthalmol 59:773–783

Murube del Castillo J, Martinez Baradas A, Hernandez King J, Cruz Vilella ME, Bahamon Caycedo M (1992) Dacryo-fornix-rhinostomy with two flaps. Eur J Ophthalmol 2:73–78

Nissen JN, Sorensen T (1987) Conjunctivorhinostomy: a study of 21 cases. Acta Ophthalmol 65:30–37

Patel BCK, Anderson R (2000) Silicone intubation in adults and children. In: Mauriello JA Jr (ed) Unfavorable results of eyelid and lacrimal surgery. Butterworth-Heinemann, Oxford, pp 491–503

Sham CL, van Hasselt CA (2000) Endoscopic terminal dacryocystorhinostomy. Laryngoscope 110:1045–1049

Soll DB (1983) Vein grafting in nasolacrimal system reconstruction. Ophthalmic Surg 14:656–662

Struck HG, Tost F (1999) Postoperative complications of Toti DCR. An indication for canalicular surgery. Ophthalmologe 96:443–447

Walter C (1997) Tränenwegstraumen. In: Walter C (ed) Plastisch-chirurgische Eingriffe im Kopf-Hals-Bereich. Thieme, Stuttgart, pp 66–67

Weidenbecher M, Hosemann W, Buhr W (1994) Endoscopic endonasal dacryocystorhinostomy: results in 56 patients. Ann Otol Rhinol Laryngol 103:363–367

Welham RA, Wulc AE (1987) Management of unsuccessful lacrimal surgery. Br J Ophthalmol 71:152–157

Yung MW, Hardman-Lea S (2003) Ipswich lacrimal tube: pedicle nasal septal tube for the reconstruction of lacrimal drainage passage. J Laryngol Otol 117:130–131

Chapter 12

Conjunctivodacryocystorhinostomy with the Insertion of a Jones Tube

12

P. Komínek

Core Messages

- Conjunctivodacryocystorhinostomy (CDCR) with the insertion of a bypass tube is a procedure in which a new lacrimal route from the conjunctival sac into the nasal cavity is created and a drainage tube is inserted between the inner canthus and the nasal cavity.
- The CDCR is carried out only in the canalicular obstructions if there is not any other surgical procedure available.
- Despite that minimally 50–60% of patients require replacing a tube within 5 years, the success rate of the procedure varies from 80 to 90%.
- The best thing seems to be Pyrex glass tube, which is used most commonly.
- The tube is considered a life-long prosthesis. If a Jones tube is extruded or lost, the recurrence of symptoms and the opening of the closure can be observed in the course of a few days because of the tunnel's non-functioning.

Contents

12.1 Introduction

Conjunctivodacryocystorhinostomy (CDCR) with the insertion of a bypass tube (Table 12.1) is a procedure in which a new lacrimal route from the conjunctival sac into the nasal cavity is created and a drainage tube is inserted between the inner canthus and the nasal cavity (Fig. 12.1). The tube in place is considered a life-long prosthesis. The procedure is mostly indicated if the upper and lower ipsilateral canaliculi are completely obstructed [11, 23]. The success rate of the procedure varies from 80 to 90% [24].

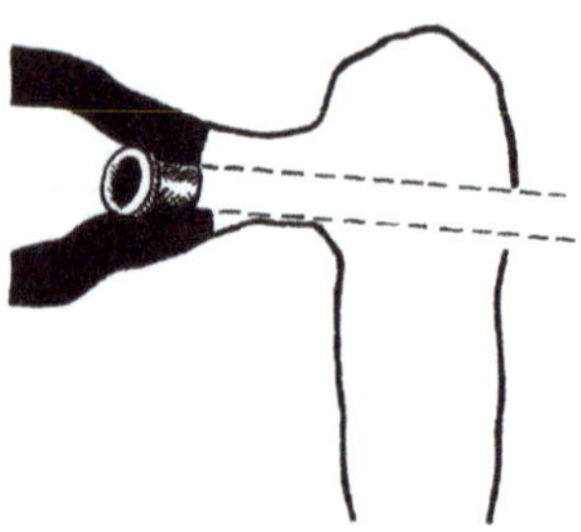

Fig. 12.1. Total lower and upper canalicular obstructions with Jones tube insertion. (From [14])

Table 12.1. Conjunctivocystorhinostomy with bypass tube

Tube placement (timing)
Primary placement (extensive canalicular obstruction)
With external DCR (EXT-DCR)
With endonasal DCR (EDCR)
Secondary placement (after failed canalicular surgery with DCR)
Closed placement with endonasal monitoring after failed DCR
Tube replacement
Location of the tube
Precanalicularly (caruncle)
Transcanalicularly (lower eyelid, medial to the punctum)

The canalicular obstructions, especially a proximal canalicular obstruction, represent a problematic and therapeutically the most difficult part of lacrimal surgery. In the medial canalicular obstructions and/or common canaliculus obstructions, a proximal patent part of canaliculi can be used for the lacrimal system reconstruction, e.g., canaliculodacryocystorhinostomy; however, it is usually not possible to use canaliculi for the reconstruction in proximal canalicular or complete canalicular obstructions. Many attempts have been made for the relief of the proximal canalicular or extensive canalicular obstructions (see Table 11.2) to produce an epithelial lined tract between the conjunctival sac and the lacrimal sac and nasal cavity, ethmoidal, or antral sinus [11, 21]. The conjunctival flaps have been pulled towards the lacrimal sac and/or the mucosa or grafts of veins have been pulled towards the conjunctiva and/or grafts of veins or the mucosa has been used. Those operations were called lacodacryostomy, lacoductostomy, conjuctivorhinostomy, conjunctivocystorhinostomy, or conjunctivodacryocystorhinostomy, and at present they are rarely performed (Fig. 12.2). The main disadvantage of those techniques is, despite this new epi-

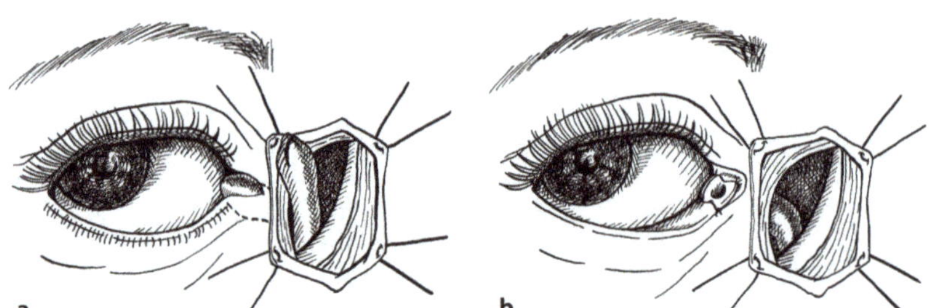

Fig. 12.2. Transposition of a lacrimal sac in a canalicular obstruction. a External conjunctivocystorhinostomy with the transposition of lacrimal sac. b Lacrimal sac is fixed in the medial canthus. (From [14])

Table 12.2. Etiology of extensive canalicular obstructions

Canalicular trauma
Radiotherapy
Congenital punctal and canalicular agenesis
Infections (herpes simplex zoster, chlamydia, trachoma, etc.)
Cytostatic therapy (5-fluorouracil)
Following medial canthal tumor excision with extirpation of lacrimal system
Following failed canalicular and other lacrimal surgery
Idiopathic

thelial-lined tract opened for syringing, the patients are not usually free of epiphora due to non-functioning of the lacrimal pump [21].

A glass bypass tube between the conjunctival sac and the nasal cavity was used for the first time in 1925 by J. Heermann, a German otorhinolaryngologist. The tube was inserted through the lower canaliculus [4, 9]. In the ophthalmology literature this procedure is connected with the name of Lester Jones, who described the surgery in 1962. While Heermann used an endonasal approach for the procedure, Jones used an external approach and this technique has prevailed for many years. The procedure is known as Jones' conjunctivodacryocystorhinostomy or dacryocystorhinostomy + bypass tube, conjunctive dacryocystorhinostomy, or dacryocystorhinostomy + Jones tube [11–14].

The renaissance of endonasal approach has been widely accepted for lacrimal surgery since the 1980s with the advent of new instruments: rigid fiberoptic endoscope and techniques for endoscopic sinus surgery, with which the procedures can be performed easily and safely. The nasal endoscopy in CDCR enables to perform dacryocystorhinostomy, placement of a tube, and adjunctive intranasal procedures such as a middle turbinectomy or septoplasty. Endoscopy is helpful in the maintenance of a tube, which is often the most challenging and critical aspect of the procedure. The choice of endoscopic vs external CDCR, however, remains that of the lacrimal surgeon guided by his or her surgical experience and the specific surgical case at hand [27].

12.2 Indications and Contraindications

12.2.1 Indications

The following indications are in effect:

1. Less than 8 mm of patent canaliculus from punctum, i.e., an extensive proximal canalicular obstrucion, acquired or congenital, that cannot be used for a canalicular reconstruction. The agenesis of lacrimal punctum with no punctal papillae can be included in this group because of non-developing or maldeveloping the canaliculi and the sac.
2. Severe trauma to the upper and lower canaliculi proximally. Attempts to reconstruct canalicular lacerations have failed.
3. Failed canaliculodacryocystorhinostomy or other canalicular surgery.
4. Severe canalicular stenoses.
5. Tumors of the inner canthi following dacryocystectomy and canaliculectomy.

12.2.2 Contraindications

The following contraindications are in effect:

1. Patency of the lacrimal system is a principal contraindication for the placement of a bypass tube; however, in severe canalicular stenosis CDCR can be the only effective procedure.
2. Lid malposition is a relative contraindication. A reconstruction of the traumatic eyelid malposition is supposed prior to Jones tube placement. The proper eyelid closure is important, not only for drainage function but also for the fixation of a tube. If there is an orbicularis weakness, e.g., in patients with facial nerve palsy, the performance of surgery is expected to be much worse due to non-functioning of the lacrimal pump and orbicularis. It is because the effect of blinking and lid functioning for drainage function with a bypass tube is fundamental. According to our experience, it is better to make the indication in those patients very carefully.

3. Age of patient is a relative contraindication for reasons of postoperative care and poorer cooperation in small children [24]. We assume the lowest age for the procedure to be 12 years.

12.3 Case History

Canalicular infections and a trauma of the eyelids and medial canthal area are typical causes of the canalicular obstruction. Canalicular obstructions can also appear following radiotherapy, systemic cytostatic therapy, etc. The cause of canalicular obstructions, however, is not often revealed and stenosis or complete obstruction is often found without etiological determination [11, 24].

There are a lot of surgical procedures and surgical modalities used in the therapy of the canalicular obstructions, e.g., laser canaliculoplasty, DCR, CDCR, canaliculocystorhinostomy, silicone intubation, etc. A choice of the optimal procedure depends on the location of the obstruction, its length, and the length of the proximal patent part of canaliculi. Their determination is an essential diagnostic problem [7].

A CDCR is to be performed if the upper and lower ipsilateral canaliculi are completely obstructed. While it is no problem to measure the length of proximal patent part from the punctum to the obstruction with simple probing, it is difficult to determine the status of canaliculus distal to the obstruction. It can be guided only by probing and exploration with retrograde probing via the common canalicular opening; however, the external approach is required and it is not easy to perform it in practice [22]. A dacryocystography and retrograde canaliculography with the injection of the contrast medium into the lacrimal sac can be used, but only theoretically. In addition, the results of canalicular surgery in proximal obstructions are controversial, and that is why a CDCR with a Jones tube placement is mostly preferred in proximal canalicular obstructions [11].

12.4 Nasal Examination

The nasal examination should be performed prior to lacrimal surgery to prevent potential problems [22, 30]. It is important especially prior to a CDCR with the external approach, because there it can be difficult to solve unexpected intranasal problems during the operation, e.g., bleeding.

There are some anatomical findings which can lead to a drainage failure: middle turbinate position and significant septal deviation. Limited turbinectomy (resection of the anterior part of the middle turbinate) is to be performed by otorhinolaryngologist in all CDCRs to prevent tube dislocation and its obstruction with the nasal mucosa. Septoplasty should be performed in significant septal deviation and/or if some problems after surgery are expected [22, 29]. If the endonasal approach is used for a DCR prior to a tube-closed placement, the partial turbinectomy is performed by otorhinolaryngologists in one sitting.

12.5 Instrumentation: Drainage Bypass Tubes

Tubes of different materials have been used for the procedure (polyethylene, silicone, Teflon, polypropylene, and glass). The materials of tubes should be of some special qualities, i.e., they should not be porous and hydrophobic and must have some rigidity so that they do not collapse and no reaction in the surrounding tissues causes arises. The best thing seems to be Pyrex glass tube, which is used most commonly (Fig. 12.3). We have our personal experience with silicone and glass tubes, and we found the latter much more convenient (Weiss Scientific Glass Blowing Co., Portland, Ore.).

Tubes can be straight or curved. Better drainage is along a straight tube than a curved tube, which is supposed to reduce the tube migration and improve positioning. Pyrex glass tubes have ocular flanges, measuring 3.0, 3.5, and 4.0 mm, and the tubes have a gentle nasal flange. The outer diameter is 2.5 mm along the shaft of the tube and inner diameter is 1.5–1.7 mm. The length of the tubes varies from 9 to 25 mm. The straight tubes 14–17 mm long are used most commonly according to our experience.

The stability of a tube is insured with an ocular and a nasal flanges. It prevents the tube from migration medially; at the nasal end, the tube gradually flares to a 2.8-mm diameter, which prevents lateral displacement of the tube [23]. Nevertheless, the extrusion of the tube is a common complication [11, 20]. To prevent migration, the tubes with small suture holes at the junction of the head and neck of a tube can be used. Glastone and Putterman reported using

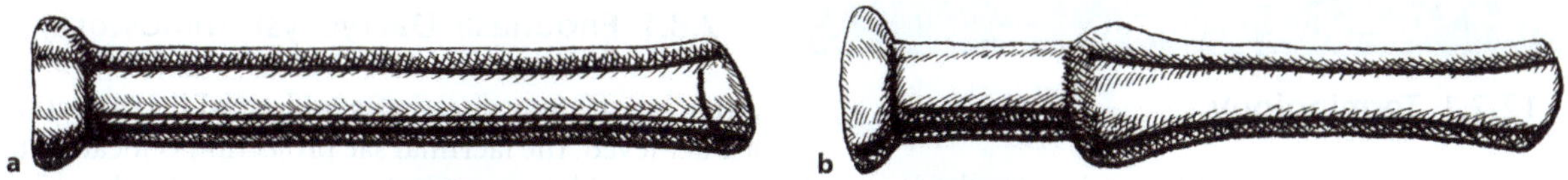

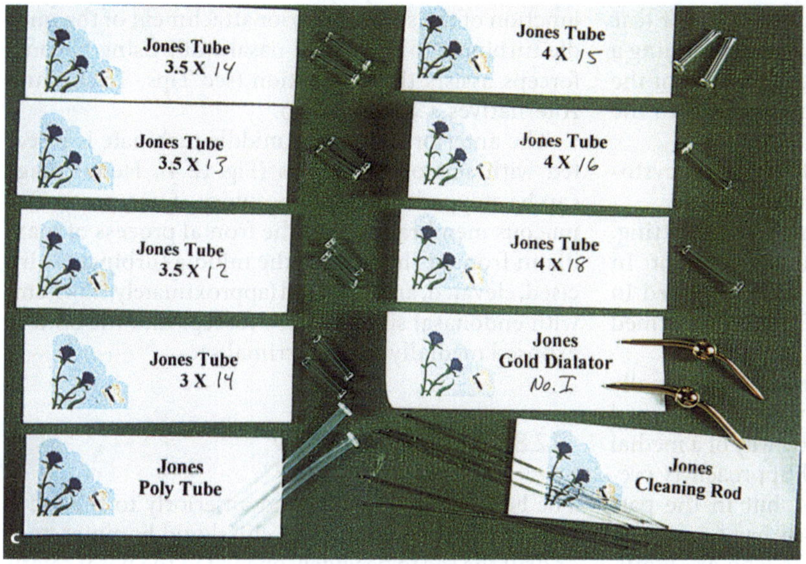

Fig. 12.3. a Standard straight glass Jones tube with an ocular flange. b Modified tube with an ocular flange and the other flange 5 mm from the top. c Jones glass Pyrex tubes. It is important to have prior surgery tubes of different length. (From [14])

of the tube with a flange in the middle of the tube, which helps to stabilize a tube [6, 20, 23]. The modified tube has another flange, measuring 3.2 mm placed 3–6 mm from the top flange.

12.6 Anesthesia

A CDCR can be performed under general anesthesia or under local anesthesia with or without any sedation. We prefer general anesthesia with tracheal intubation in all patients under the perfect airway control, not only in young, uncooperative, nervous, and anxious patients. General anesthesia allows a peaceful performance of the procedure, which is comfortable for the patient and the surgeon as well. It is important in all procedures that can be complicated with bleeding, which is usually the major problem, and it concerns a CDCR as well. The modern medications used for general anesthesia provide safe conduct of anesthesia and surgery without or with a minimum of postoperative side effects.

Bleeding is the major complication in a CDCR. To decrease this complication, the vasoconstriction of the nasal mucosa is performed. As the procedure is performed similarly to the other endonasal sinus procedures, the vasoconstriction is performed in the same way:

1. A nasal spray or drops of oxymetazolin is used preoperatively. Before the surgery, two applications of 0.1% solution are administered to the nasal cavity during a half an hour.
2. The pledglets soaked with 1:10,000 epinephrin (2–5 ml) are placed in the nasal cavity shortly after intubation.
3. The lateral nasal wall and middle turbinate are injected with 2–4 ml of 1% trimecain + 1:100,000 epinephrin and the pledges soaked with 1:10,000 epinephrin are placed in the nasal cavity again. After satisfactory anesthesia and nasal decongestion are achieved, i.e., after 5–10 min, the operation starts.

12.7 Operative Technique

12.7.1 Terminology

The main aim of a CDCR is to bypass the lacrimal system altogether and to create a new conduit for tear outflow [22, 27]. This is done by careful positioning a small tube between the tear lake at the region of the caruncle and the middle meatus just anterior to the middle turbinate [27].

The procedure consists of two steps: dacryocystorhinostomy (DCR) and tube placement.

If both of those steps are performed in one sitting, the tube placement is called primary placement. In the secondary closed placement, a tube is placed in the separate sitting, whereas the DCR is performed prior the placement.

A CDCR with Jones tube placement as originally described by Jones has traditionally been performed as an "open" or external procedure by way of a medial canthal incision [27]. The external approach is preferred mostly by ophthalmologists, but in the past two decades the endonasal approach has been more frequently by otorhinolaryngologists who are familiar with endonasal sinus surgery [14, 22]. The endonasal approach is especially advantageous in secondary tube placement after failed canalicular surgery with DCR, in which a bone window had been done [27].

The tube can be placed precanalicularly (caruncle) or transcanalicularly (lower eyelid, medial to the punctum). The medial canthal or caruncle placement is used more often. It is usually necessary to remove part of the caruncle; however, the stability of a tube is better and a shorter tube is used. The transcanalicular placement can be used if there is a wide lower punctum. A tube is placed in the posterior lamella of the eyelid [24]; however, it is important to use a longer tube and there is a greater tendency for the tube to fall out [22].

12.8 Primary CDCR with Jones Tube with Endonasal Approach

The procedure consists of two steps: endonasal dacryocystorhinostomy and tube placement.

12.8.1 Endonasal Dacryocystorhinostomy

After satisfactory anesthesia and nasal decongestion are achieved, the lacrimal sac projection is located intranasally. The sac projection is expected to be at the junction of the superoanterior attachment of the middle turbinate to the lateral nasal wall. Using bayonet forceps assists the orientation (see Tips, Tricks, and Alternatives, Chapter 12.11).

The anterior part of the middle turbinate is resected with scissor or forceps (Fig. 12.4). Hemorrhage can be stopped with electrocautery, if necessary. The mucous membrane above the frontal process of maxilla in front of the head of the middle turbinate is incised, elevated, and removed (approximately 1.5×1 cm) with endonasal sinus surgery forceps and the bone is exposed medially to the lacrimal sac.

12.8.1.1 Bone Window

The bone lying medially and anteriorly to the sac is mostly removed with using chisel and hammer and/or drill the sac to be widely opened to the nasal cavity. The anterior ethmoid cells have to be removed in some cases to achieve it, too.

It is important that the bone window be wide enough for the bone not to push later on a glass tube. If a surgical drill is used for a bone removal, care must be taken not to cause a zone of bone necrosis. So, simultaneously irrigation and suction must be done. The edges of the bone window can be palpated in the medial canthus from the outside. If the bone window is not wide enough, especially in the inferomedial direction, it must be widened and a tube can be then inserted.

12.8.1.2 Sac Opening

The sac is incised with a sickle knife and opened and the medial wall of the sac is removed or the mucosal flap of the lacrimal sac can sometimes be placed posteriorly to keep the sac widely opened.

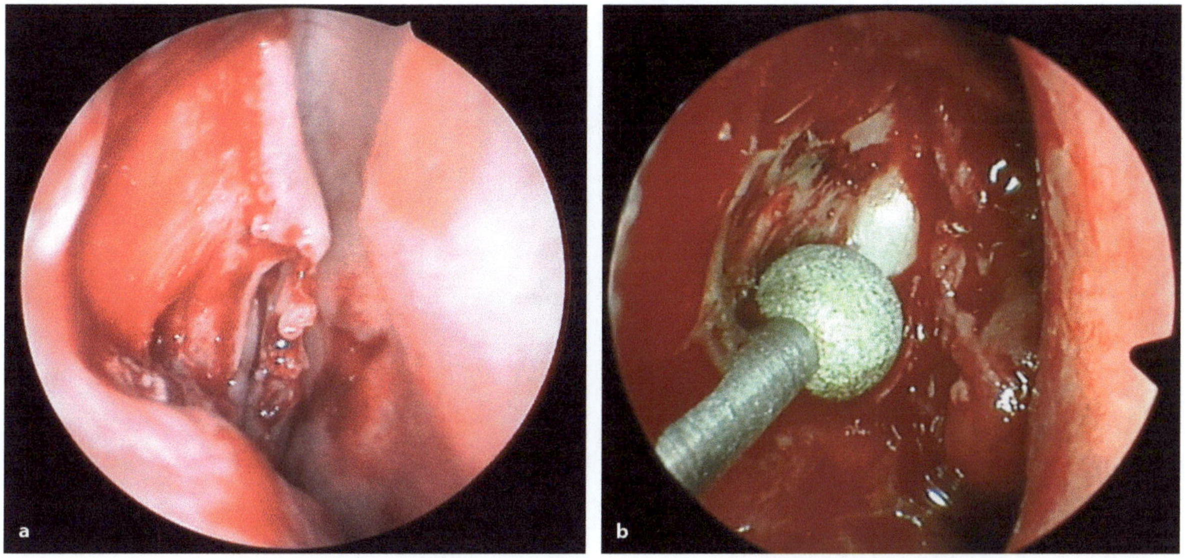

Fig. 12.4. Dacryocystorhinostomy is carried out as an initial part of the procedure. It can be performed from the endonasal or external approach. **a** Removal of anterior portion of middle concha (*right*) prevents postoperative complications. **b** The bone is removed with the help of drill (shown), chisel, or laser

12.8.2 Tube Placement

The following steps are taken for tube placement:

1. Caruncle bipolar electrocautery is performed prior the tube placement to reduce the caruncle (Fig. 12.5). It gives a better access to the entry at the medial canthus. Electrocautery is preferred to cutting a caruncle because it makes hemostasis, and the conjunctiva has a less tendency to cover later the tube.
2. A needle (or a guide wire) is passed in the medial canthus from the site of the caruncle (or anterior/inferior caruncle) into the nasal cavity in the inferomedial direction. Viewing endonasally with Hopkins endoscope can confirm that the needle positioning is correct and the length of the tunnel can be measured.
3. The tunnel is cut with the help of a Graefe knife along a needle into the nasal cavity through the soft tissues while the cornea is preserved with a protector (Fig. 12.6). The opening of the tunnel can be enlarged with moving the knife inferiorly and then superiorly, if necessary (the knife end is pushed and pulled with short movements in superior and inferior directions to enlarge the track) and its intranasal positioning can be confirmed endoscopically.

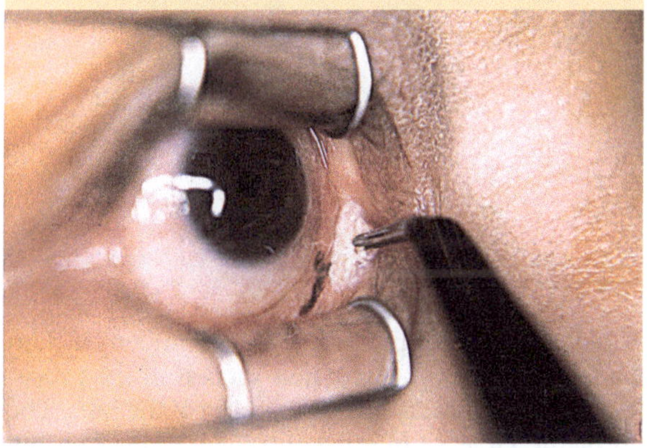

Fig. 12.5. Electrocautery of the caruncle gives good access to the entry at the medial canthus. (From [14])

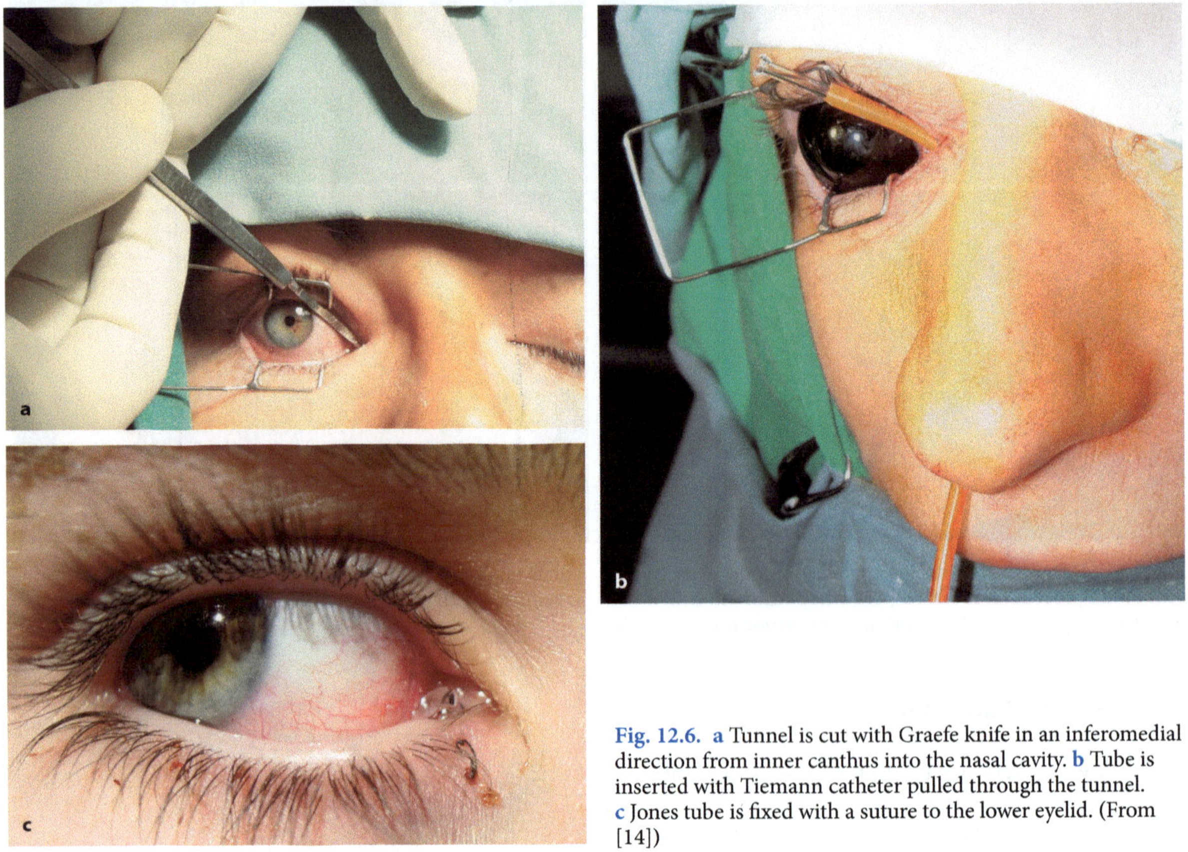

Fig. 12.6. a Tunnel is cut with Graefe knife in an inferomedial direction from inner canthus into the nasal cavity. b Tube is inserted with Tiemann catheter pulled through the tunnel. c Jones tube is fixed with a suture to the lower eyelid. (From [14])

12.8.2.1 Length of a Tube

A tube should be approximately 2–4 mm longer than the length of a tunnel, because success of the procedure depends on accurate positioning of the tube. The tip of the Graefe knife is controlled endoscopically to be 2–4 mm over the lateral nasal wall and the edge of the knife is grasped at the medial canthus with a hemostat of tweezers and the Graefe knife is then withrawn. This process provides a measure of the distance from the medial canthus to the knife tip and the determination of an appropriate length of the tube [20].

11.8.2.2 Tube Insertion

A tube is inserted with the help of Thiemann urological catheter, the outer diameter of 8 Charrier, or with a guide wire. A Jones tube is put into the luminous end of Thiemann catheter not farther than 2 mm. The catheter tip is put into the cut tunnel from the caruncle and the catheter placement is controlled endonasally with endoscope. The tip is caught with forceps and pulled out of the nose and thus a glass tube is gently inserted into the tunnel. At this moment the flange of the tube is fixed with forceps in the medial canthus and the catheter is drawn out of the tube. The correct placement of a tube and its length are controlled endoscopically.

12.8.2.3 Tube Fixation

The tube is fixed with a Prolene suture 8-0 around its neck to the medial part of the lower eyelid. The suture is removed in 4–6 weeks. A Jones tube with a hole at the neck makes suturing easier.

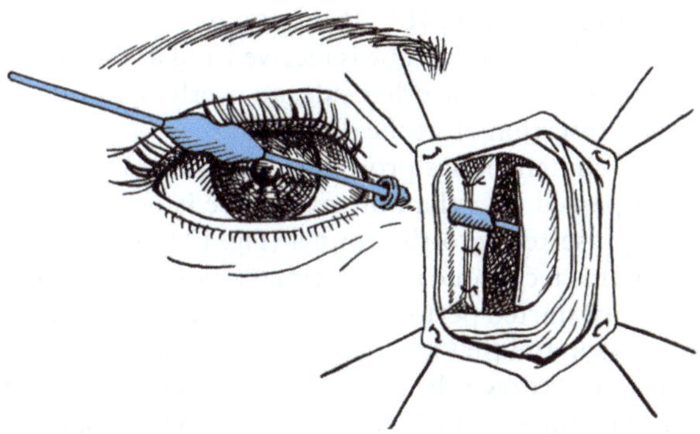

Fig. 12.7. The CDCR with an external approach. Tube is inserted into the tunnel after the posterior nasal and lacrimal sac flaps were anastomosed. (From [14])

12.9 External vs Closed Approach

Most reports of CDCRs have described an external approach (Fig. 12.7) [28].

The primary CDCR with external tube placement starts with a standard DCR with the incision on the side of the nose. The tube is placed after posterior lacrimal sac and nasal flaps are anastomosed. If the tube position is definitely good, the anterior lacrimal and nasal flaps are sutured [11–13].

The endoscopic closed CDCRs have been also performed in past years because endoscopic visualization is critical in the placement of the Jones tube [22, 27, 28]. The advantages of endoscopic CDCR are the same as those cited for DCR, i.e., lack of cutaneous scar, shorter operation time, and blood loss [7, 28]. An endoscopic approach allows the surgeon excellent intranasal visualization to perform a middle turbinate resection and to assess the proper length and positioning of the tube. The technique for endonasal surgery is much more expensive than the equipment for a traditional external CDCR; however, this fact has lost its importance because the equipment necessary for endoscopic CDCR is now readily available in most hospitals and ambulatory surgery centers [27]. That is why an endonasal approach is used more frequently than it was 20 years ago.

As in the revision DCR, the endoscopic approach is favourable in the setting of a revisions procedure, i.e., in secondary tube placement, which provides superior intranasal visualization [11, 22, 27, 28]. The choice of external or endonasal endoscopic CDCR remains up to the lacrimal surgeon, guided by surgical experience [28].

12.10 Secondary Tube Placement

The secondary tube placement is performed if DCR failed and with canalicular surgery. The tube placement is easier to perform because of less hemorrhage and more consistent (solid) tissues between the medial canthus and nasal cavity following surgery and the bone window was carried out in previous surgery. A tube can be placed if the bone window has been made wide enough for the tunnel to be performed.

The procedure is performed under general or local anesthesia and the tube is placed in the same manner as the primary procedure.

12.11 Tips, Tricks, and Alternatives

There are some points which can make some troubles in the procedures, especially tube insertion and tube stability, which can be influenced by many factors such as the distension of the tunnel, its direction, choice of the tube, its fixation, etc.

12.11.1 Lacrimal Sac Location

The lacrimal sac cannot be located with the help of transcanalicular translumination due to the canalicular obstruction. That is why the intranasal orientation during the procedure need not be easy, especially for beginners.

Using nasal bayonet forceps is useful for the orientation in locating a lacrimal sac projection (Fig. 12.8). One jaw of the forceps is placed extranasally and held in the medial canthus. The other jaw placed intranasally accords with the lacrimal sac projection on the lateral nasal wall and indicates the place to look for the lacrimal sac. This procedure can be easily repeated during the surgery [17].

12.11.2 Direction of the Tunnel

It is advisable to direct the tube in the infero-medial direction, i.e., 30–45% inferiorly. If the tube is hori-

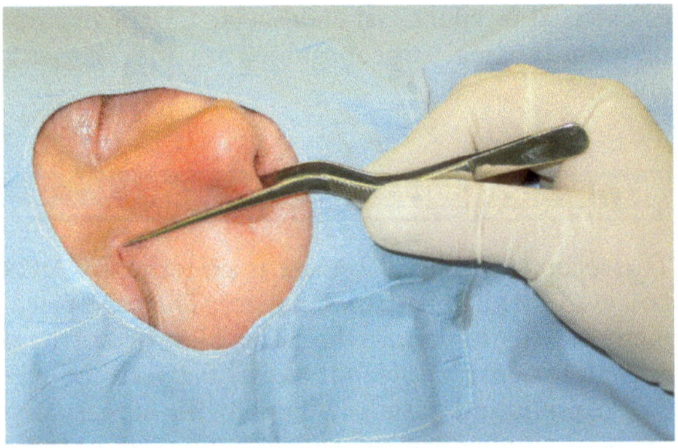

Fig. 12.8. Lacrimal sac location. Intranasal orientation is easier with bayonet forceps to locate lacrimal sac projection. One jaw is held in the medial canthus. The other jaw placed intranasally accords with the lacrimal sac projection on the lateral nasal wall

zontal, its stability is worse and there is a higher risk of tube extrusion. The inferomedial direction is important for the drainage function because gravitation plays an important role in tear drainage [21, 24].

12.11.3 Insertion of the Tube

Tunnel should be appropriately wide so that the fit between the tube and the tunnel should minimize postoperative extrusion [10]. If the tunnel is too wide, a worse stability of the tube is received and its extrusion is supposed. On the other side, an overly tight tunnel makes insertion of a tube difficult.

In standard Jones procedure a bypass tube placement passed over the Bowman probe is described as being inserted into the tunnel (Fig. 12.9a). We were using this technique in the primary closed placement when we started performing CDCR procedures; however, we found that it had been difficult sometimes to place a tube down the tunnel because the nasal end of the glass tube is a little wider than the outer diameter and often draws up soft tissues of the tunnel in front of it and makes placing more complicated. In spite of using the Bowman probe or Kirschner wire, tube insertion can be very stressful. In those cases the tube insertion can be achieved by slight traction on the margins of the opening or the tube is aided by rotation of it with forceps or by widening the tunnel; however, it can cause tube migration and its loss. [10].

The troubles with the tube insertion were the reason for using the Thiemann urological catheter [16]. The Tiemann cathether tip is slightly hooked, ball shaped, fluently extended in its diameter, is sufficiently hard (but not as much as the wire), and it enables distension of the tunnel, which need not be too wide.

A similar principle of the tube placement uses vessel dilator recommended by Gonnering [7, 8, 22]. The vessel dilator is cut 4 cm from its distal end and

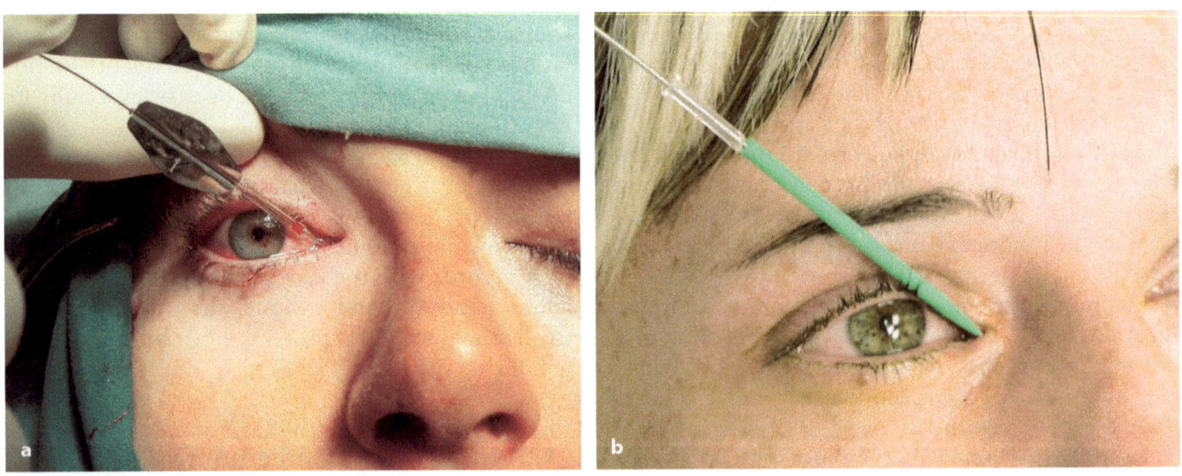

Fig. 12.9. a Closed tube insertion of Jones tube placed over Bowman probe. If the tunnel is appropriately wide, the tube insertion can be achieved by slight traction on the margins of the opening or the tube being rotated with forceps. b Tube insertion with vessel dilator. Tube is placed over a guide wire

threaded over the guide wire and the Jones tube is threaded on the guide wire behind the dilator segment [8]. The dilator ahead of the Jones tube is confirmed intranasally and the Jones tube is placed into the tunnel tightly behind the dilator (Fig. 12.9b). The vessel dilator and guide wire are then both removed from the nostril [8]. We have experience only with a few procedures performed in this manner.

The trephine, described by Henderson, can achieve optimal tunnel to make the tube placement accurate [10]. A core of the soft tissues is cut with the trephine and the tube is introduced on the guide wire so that it enables better positioning and stability of the tube [10, 22]. We do not have experience with this technique.

If a wire is passed transcanalicularly, it is passed into the nose from the lower canalicular ampulla (opened by a three-snip procedure).

12.11.4 Length of the Tube

The tube must not be either very long nor very short. A long tube may extrude proximally and the nasal lumen can be obstructed with the mucosa of the septum or the turbinate. A short tube can be overgrowth with the nasal mucosa especially if it migrates laterally.

The distal nasal end should be 2–4 mm over the nasal wall, minimally 2–3 mm from the septal mucosa [11, 19, 24]. An optimal tube can be replaced later, if necessary; endonasal telescope assists in the visualization and correct positioning.

12.11.5 Fixation of the Tube

The fixation of a tube with a suture around its collar significantly decreases a risk of its extrusion and loss [19, 23]. Since we started to do it, the extrusion rate and migration have been observed less frequently. Can observed less extrusion after insertion of the Jones tube circumscribed with a buccal mucosa graft [2].

12.11.6 Nasal Pathology

Nasal pathology, including septal deviation and impacted middle turbinates, are factors in failures with the Jones tube [29, 30]. These conditions can be handled prior to the insertion of the tube, if recognized. An otolaryngological consultation should be performed and surgery on the nose, if indicated, should be done prior to the insertion of the CDCR.

If there is a significant septal deviation, it is better to perform septoplasty prior the lacrimal surgery [30]. If we hesitate, we recommend doing it, according to our experience, to avoid postoperative problems.

The anterior tip of the middle turbinate is sometimes found to obstruct the inner end of a tube. If the middle turbinate is allowed to remain in place, contact with the glass tube can cause bleeding, discharge, and pain. The tube may change its position, irritating the eye, and ceasing to function [29]. We recommend to perform the resection of the anterior tip of the middle turbinate in all CDCRs because it decreases postoperative complications.

12.12 Highlights

The CDCRs have their limits and not all patients with canalicular obstruction are suitable candidates for surgery. The tube placement is permanent, i.e., a long-life prosthesis. It differs significantly from a temporary silicone intubation in DCR or canaliculocystorhinostomy. If a Jones tube is extruded or lost, the recurrence of symptoms and the opening closure can be observed in the course of a few days because of the tunnel's not functioning. There are only rare cases in which the opening may be left open and the patients are free of symptoms.

A DCR is a highly successful procedure, especially in patients 20–69 years [25]. A reported success rate of Jones tube placement with relief of epiphora varies between 41 and 100% (according to experience, it is 85–90%) [7, 14]; however, a high success rate is associated with a significant number of complications, much higher than after DCR. [2, 3, 11, 14, 22, 24]. That is why a postoperative follow-up period may in fact require more than one surgical procedure to reach that point. In addition, 15–20% of the patients are expected not to be satisfied with the results despite the good functioning of the procedure. The postoperative care and the number of follow-up examinations, tube maintenance, fogging and spraying of spectacles, and discomfort may contribute to a patient's satisfaction despite a completely dry eye [18]. The patients have to be informed preoperatively that CDCR cannot guarantee a comfortable, dry eye, and that a lot of complications can occur in tube maintenance in the long term is necessary [11, 25]. It can prevent their dissatisfaction and frustration.

That is why very good motivation and good cooperation are the basic conditions for the surgery. It is important to discuss all alternatives with a patient before the procedure and again immediately after the surgery to explain the nature of the operation, its goal, and limitations and the commitment to a long period of frequent postoperative follow-up examination [11, 18, 25]. The patients must be prepared for a possibility of secondary surgery. This explanation may reduce dissatisfaction resulting from overly high expectations [24].

12.13 Postoperative Care and Complications

12.13.1 Postoperative Care

12.13.1.1 The Follow-up Examination

It is advisable to perform examinations 1 week, 1 months, 3 months, and 6 months after surgery and later minimally once a year. [18]. The patients are recommended to return for a review if problems with the tube occurs.

12

The examination includes an inspection of a position of the tube, fluorescein dye disappearance test, the sniff test (see below), and endonasal endoscopy. The postoperative function can be evaluated by using a FDT viewed directly (Fig. 12.10). Endonasal endoscopy is fast and efficient and facilitates the maintenance of a tube function with a minimal manipulation and patient discomfort, including a inspection of the length and a position of the glass tube [1]. That is why close cooperation between ophthalmologists and otorhinolaryngologists is needed.

12.13.1.2 Care Immediately After Surgery

Applying steroid-antibiotic drops is recommended for 1 week. The patients are recommended to wet their nose with sprays and lavages. They should not blow the nose for 4–5 days, and only if necessary, and only very gently, because emphysema can occur. Patients are allowed to blow the nose later; however, to prevent the tube extrusion (Table 11.3), the tube must be protected with holding a finger over the medial canthus and/or the patient must close the eyes tightly. It is important to show it to the patients and to explain it and check if they know how to do it. Patients must be instructed not to wipe their eyes but only pat them towards the nose to avoid a extrusion of the tube.

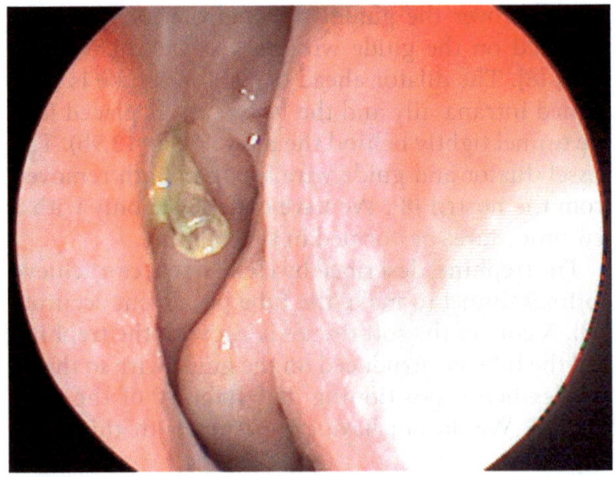

Fig. 12.10. Nasal cavity and the proper tube position a few weeks after surgery (*right*)

Table 12.3. Prevention of tube extrusion

Interomedial direction of the tunnel (tube)
The tunnel is not to be very wide
Suturing of a tube with the skin (eyelid)
Puttermann modified tubes with a double flange
Blowing one's nose with closed eyelid or with a finger over the medial canthus
Angled glass tubes

12.13.1.3 Cleaning a Tube

A tube has to be cleaned every day in the morning to be patent. Tube maintenance is often the most challenging and critical aspects of CDCR. The tube is cleaned with the sniff test: the patient is told to splash some water in the conjunctival sac, to hold the other nostril, and to sniff (snort) water from the medial canthus into the tube and the nose. The air and water pass down the tube, and this rash can be acoustically noticed by the patient (sniff test).

12.13.1.4 Blowing One's Nose

As there is a greater risk of lateral tube migration and loss, it is not recommended to blow the nose without closed eyelids or holding the tube with a finger. It is important to check the patient's ability to perform this maneuver at visits. Sometimes the tube can be plugged with a lot of mucous discharge. Some decongestant eyedrops can be used and the tube cleaned with the same technique. Some patients would be able to clean the tube with a probe, if necessary, but we do not recommend it.

12.13.2 Complications

12.13.2.1 Extrusion of the Tube

One of the most frequent complications is an extrusion of the tube, which can happen in many patients [18, 24]. Minimally 50–60% of patients require replacement of a tube within 5 years [11, 14, 22].

An extrusion may occur immediately following surgery, however, in postoperative surgery it does not occur very often despite the fact that the tunnel and some fibrous tissue stabilize the tube and hold it in place.

Hypermobility of the Jones tube can be prevented in the immediate postoperative period by suturing the tube in place at the time of surgery with a 6-0 nonabsorbable suture wrapped several times around the tube near the collar [20]. The suture is left in place for 3 weeks while the tissue contracts around the tube (Fig. 12.6c). The modified tube with a double-flanged tube helps to anchor the tube in the surgical passageway and reduces its hypermobility [20].

12.13.2.2 Tube Replacement

The extrusions immediately after the surgery are usually caused by the bad fixation with a suture or by a wrong position of a tube. It usually causes no problems to reinsert the tube into the tunnel under local anesthesia shortly after the extrusion.

A Weiss gold dilator or some other dilator can be used for it, too. A tube is usually put over the Bowman probe and inserted into the opening in the medial canthus and secured with a suture; however, it is not easy to dilate the tunnel and to insert a tube if the tunnel is too contracted and scarred, and it can be unpleasant and painful (Fig. 12.11). The longer the time after the extrusion, the more complicated the reinsertion. We use wire dilators and it is advantageous to monitor an optimal length of the tube and its nasal positioning with the help of an endoscope.

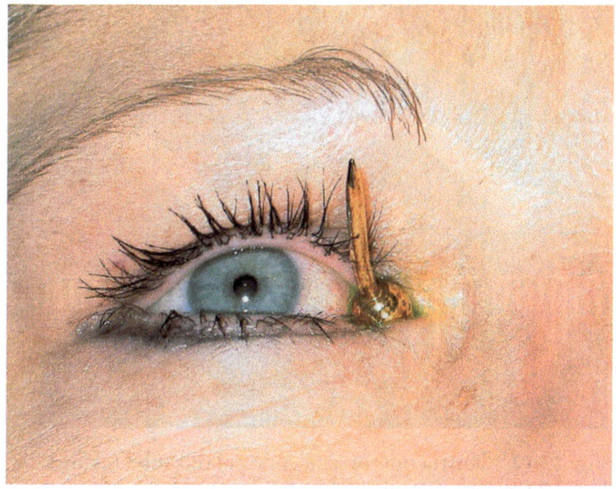

Fig. 12.11. Replacing Jones tube. Dilator opens and dilates the existing tract

12.13.2.3 Malposition (Migration) of the Tube

Migration is a common complication. There are lateral and medial migrations. Lateral migration can be observed if the septum or middle turbinate is pushing the tube laterally or it can be caused by cicatrix formation at the lateral nasal wall. It can be caused by hypertrophy of the middle turbinate, too, and the turbinectomy is usually needed if it has not been performed. We recommend to perform resection of the anterior tip of the middle turbinate in all CDCRs. Since we started fixing the tubes with a suture to the eyelid, we have seen this complication only rarely.

Medial migration usually indicates that the tube is too short. It can be removed and a slightly longer one can be substituted [7]. Medial migration is relatively common following the Jones technique in which a large track is cut, and is less common with the trephining technique [23].

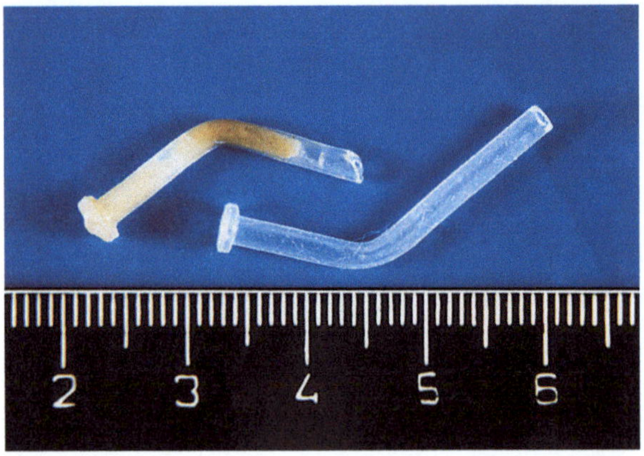

Fig. 12.12. Obstruction of a silicone curved tube (*above*), below the new one. (From [14])

12.13.2.4 Plugging the Tube

Plugging with the mucus stopper can mostly set in if the patient has not been adequately looking after the tube. It can be observed extremely rarely in patients with glass tubes and very often in patients with curved silicone tubes (Fig. 12.12). If the tube cannot be cleaned with the sniff test, it can be sometimes better to remove the tube, to clean it is carefully, and reinsert it. Obstruction of the tube by mucus plugging can be easily rectified by cleaning and syringing the tube in an outpatient setting [18].

12.13.2.5 Granulations

Granulations may be seldom formed at the ocular end of a tube coming from caruncle or conjunctiva, but they can sometimes grow over the ocular end. A small granulation can be resected with scissors under local anesthesia [30]. In some recalcitrant granulations it may be necessary to remove the tube and reinsert it after healing. We have observed such a situation only once.

The nasal end can be grown over with a granulation as well or the mucosa membrane if a tube is too short. This can be prevented with a longer tube.

12.13.2.6 End Impact

End impact on middle turbinate or septum leads to partial or total loss of function and causes intractable pain [26].

12.13.2.7 Bleeding

Bleeding after a CDCR seems to be similar to a DCR and usually causes no problems, especially for otolaryngologists who are familiar with the endonasal procedures and surgery [27]. Bleeding can be solved with the nasal packing (it is usually used at the end of the procedure), or with nasal decongestive drops. The surgeon must be careful not to push the packing on the tube at its nasal end and to push it laterally.

12.13.2.8 Breaking the Tube

Breaking the tube is theoretically possible but extremely rare. We have not observed it thus far.

12.13.2.9 Conjunctivitis

After CDCR, the conjunctival flora of the eye becomes similar to the nasal flora [3]. Conjunctivitis can be present as a result of a mild infection around the collar of the tube. It presents as a foreign body sensation and it can be treated with antibiotic steroid drops [30]. Late conjunctivitis is usually a result of scale-like deposits which have collected on the outside of a Pyrex tube and the tube should be removed and cleaned [30].

12.14 Conclusion

> A proximal canalicular obstruction can be treated with conjunctivocystorhinostomy + Jones tube placement. The procedure should be used if no other reconstruction procedures can be performed. As a high number of complications, much higher than in DCR, are observed in the postoperative period, a very good motivation should be a basic condition for successful surgery.

Reference

1. Boboridis K, Olver JM (2000) Endoscopic conjunctivodacryocystorhinostomy with Jones lacrimal bypass tubes. Opththalmic Surg Lasers 107:1206–1209
2. Can I, Can B, Yarangümeli A et al. (1999) CDCR with buccal mucosal graft: comparative and histopathological study. Ophthalmic Surg Lasers 30:98–104
3. Can I, Aribal E, Yarangümeli A et al. (1998) Changes in the conjunctival flora after conjunctivodacryocystorhinostomy (CDCR): a preliminary report. Acta J Ophthalmol 8:142–147
4. Denecke HJ, Denecke MU, Draf W et al. (1992) Die Operationen and den Nasennebenhühlen und der angrenzenden Schädelbasis. Springer, Berlin Heidelberg New York
5. Doucet TW, Hurwith JJ (1982) Canaliculodacryocystorhinostomy in the treatment of canalicular obstruction. Arch Ophthalmol 100:306–309
6. Gladstone GJ, Putterman AM (1985) A modified glass tube for conjunctivodacryocystorhinostomy. Arch Ophthalmol 103:1229–1230
7. Gonnering RS (1994) Dacryocystorhinostomy and conjunctivodacryocystorhinostomy. In: Dortzbach RK (ed) Ophthalmic plastic surgery: prevention and management of complications. Raven Press, New York, pp 237–250
8. Gonnering RS, Lyon DB, Fisher JC (1991) Endoscopic laser-assisted lacrimal surgery. Am J Ophthalmol 111:152–157
9. Heermann J (1991) Rhinochirurgische Aspekte bei Tränenwegstenosen. Otorhinolaryngol Nova 1:227–232
10. Henderson PN (1985) A modified trephine technique for the insertion of Jones tube. Arch Ophthalmol 103:1582–158
11. Hurwitz JJ (1996) The lacrimal system. Lippincott-Raven, Philadelphia
12. Jones LJ (1965) Conjunctivodacryocystorhinostomy. Am J Opthalmol 59:773–783
13. Jones LJ (1978) Conjunctive dacryocystorhinostomy. In: Yamaguchi M (ed) Recent advances on the lacrimal system. Kyoto, pp 69–70
14. Komínek P, Červenka S, Müllner K (2003) The lacrimal diseases. Diagnostics and treatment. Maxdorf, Prague
15. Komínek P, Červenka S, Matoušek P (2004) Endonasal dacryocystorhinostomy: location of lacrimal sac with forceps. Laryngoscope 114:1674–1676
16. Komínek P, Červenka S Conjunctivodacryocystorhinostomy: tube placement with the catheter. Ophthal Plast Reconstr Surg – accepted for publication
17. Lee JS, Jung G, Lewe JE et al. (2001) The treatment of lacrimal apparatus obstruction with the use of an inner canthal Jones tube insertion via a transcaruncular route. Ophthalmic Surg Lasers 32:48–54
18. Lim CH, Martin P, Benger R et al. (2004) Lacrimal canalicular bypass surgery with the Lester Jones tube. Am J Ophthalmol 137:101–108
19. McNab AA (1994) Manual of orbital and lacrimal surgery. Churchill Livingstone, Edinburgh
20. Migliori ME, Putterman AM (1989) Recurrent Jones tube extrusion successfully treated with a modified glass tube. Ophthal Plast Reconstr Surg 5:189–191
21. Murube JC (1987) External conjunctivorhinostomy. In: Smith BC (ed) Ophthalmic plastic and reconstructive surgery, vol 2. Mosby, St. Louis, pp 968–973
22. Olver J (2002) Colour atlas of lacrimal surgery. Butterworth-Heinemann, Oxford
23. Putterman AM (1988) Conjunctivodacryocystorhinostomy. In: Linberg JV (ed) Lacrimal surgery. Churchill Livingstone, New York, pp 281–296
24. Rose GE, Welham AN (1991) Jones' lacrimal canalicular bypass tubess: twenty-five years' experience. Eye 5:13–19
25. Rosen N, Ashkenazi I, Rosner M (1994) Patient dissatisfaction after functionally successful conjunctivodacryocystorhinostomy with Jones tube. Am J Ophthalmol 117:636–642
26. Sekhar DC, Dortzbach RK, Gonnering RS et al. (1991) Problems associated with conjunctivodacryocystorhinostomy. Am J Ophthalmol 112:502–506
27. Trotter WL, Meyer DR (2000) Endoscopic conjunctivodacryocystorhinostomy with Jones tube placement. Opthalmology 107:1206–1209
28. Watkins LM, Janfaza P, Tubin PA (2003) The evolution of endonasal dacryocystorhinostomy. Surv Ophthalmol 48:73–84
29. Wesley RE, Bond JB (1986) Intranasal procedures for successful lacrimal surgery. Ophthal Plast Reconstr Surg 2:153–157
30. Wobing JL (1983) Lacrimal surgery. In: Iliff NT (ed) Complications in ophthalmic surgery. Churchill Livingstone, New York, pp 371–386

Chapter 13

Interventional Radiology

13

K. Wilhelm

Core Messages

- Advances in interventional techniques in the lacrimal drainage system have expanded novel procedures for the easy and safe treatment of epiphora. These methods are simple, safe, and cost-effective, and can be performed under local anesthesia on an outpatient basis.
- Fluoroscopically guided balloon dacryocystoplasty is a feasible nonsurgical therapy in nasolacrimal duct stenosis that may be used as first-line therapy. In cases that have initial success, however, a relatively high long-term success rate can be expected.
- Stent placement should be selected with caution as a first-line therapeutic option in patients who refuse surgical procedures or are not suitable candidates for general anesthesia. Although the initial results of stent placement in patients with complete obstructions of the lacrimal drainage system are excellent, long-term results have to be improved.

Contents

13.1 Introduction

The lacrimal system has become of interest to the radiologist, as radiological interventions requiring adequate diagnostic work-up have been described. The eye doctor's patients, in whose diagnosis and treatment the radiologist may be involved, usually complain of constant tearing, epiphora. While in the past treatment of this condition was surgical (e.g., by dacryocystorhinostomy), interventional procedures have been developed and have become well established for treatment in selected cases (Song 2002).

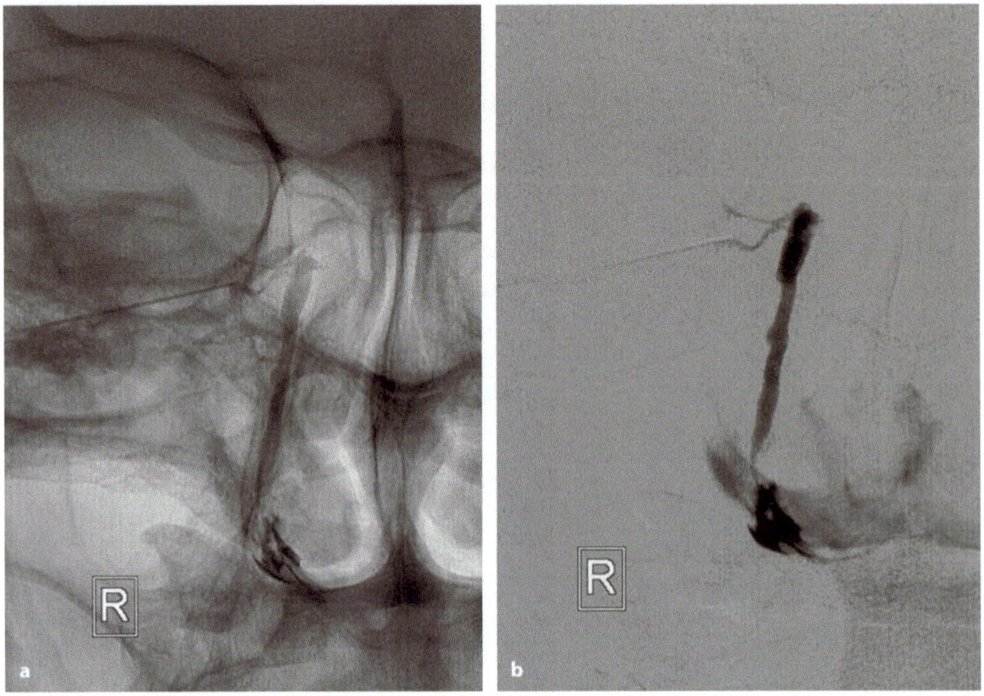

Fig. 13.1. Radiographic anatomy: dacryocystography (DCG). a Normal right DCG, frontal view, cannula in inferior canaliculus. b Digital subtracted image demonstrates patency of the canaliculi, lacrimal sac, and nasolacrimal duct. No contrast medium reflux to the eyelid is seen

13

13.2 Digital Subtraction Dacryocystography

13.2.1 Indications

To identify patients suitable for interventional therapy, the exact cause for epiphora has to be determined. When overproduction of tear fluid has been ruled out, digital subtraction dacryocystography (DCG) of the lacrimal system is performed to demonstrate obstructions of the lacrimal drainage system. The DCG is capable of determining the patency of the canaliculi, lacrimal sac, and nasolacrimal duct. When disease is present, the site and degree of obstruction or stenosis are well evaluated by DCG. Since the original description by Ewing (1989), many radiographic techniques for dacryocystography have been described. Digital subtraction dacryocystography (DSD), which combines the technique of DCG and digital subtraction fluoroscopic capabilities, has become the gold standard. The DSD is able to render high-resolution images of the complete nasolacrimal duct system. In addition, assessment of the rate of flow of contrast material yields important information regarding flow dynamics (Kassel and Schatz 1995).

13.2.2 Contraindication

The contraindication is acute inflammation of the lacrimal system.

13.2.3 Instrumentation, Anesthesia, and Operative technique

For DSD a DSA run is performed, while contrast medium (CM) is injected through a DCG catheter. To make the patient more relaxed and decrease blinking and lacrimation, it is preferred to instill a short-acting topical anesthesic into the conjunctival sac (e.g., Novesine 0.4, CIBA Vision Ophthalmics, Germering, Germany). For intubation of the lacrimal punctum, a 22 G polyvinylchloride tubing catheter (Dacryocys-

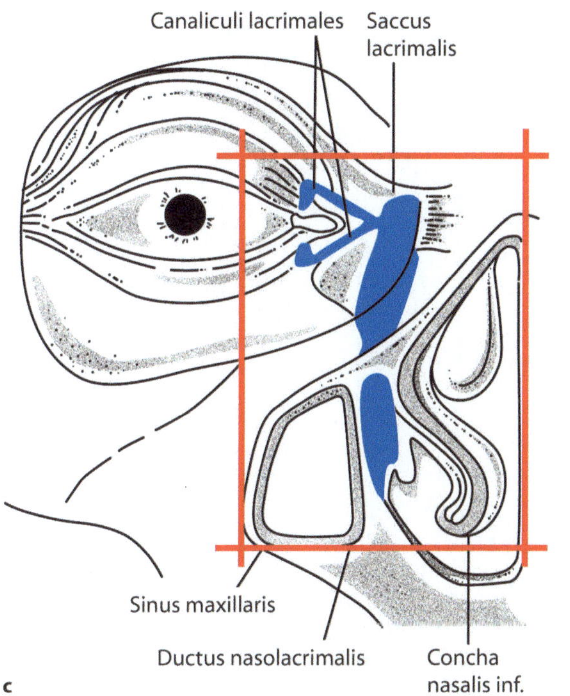

Fig. 13.1. (*Continued*) **c** Drawing of the normal anatomy of the nasolacrimal duct system (NLDS). Right eye, frontal view

tography Catheter, Cook, Queensland, Australia) is used. Water-soluble, nonionic liquid CM (Iopromide, Ultravist 300, Schering, Berlin, Germany) is injected manually during acquisition (frame rate: 2/s). In the early phase of injection, reflux can be minimized by an initial slow injection rate. Subsequently, the rate can be increased to achieve greater sac distension or to overcome resistance by partial obstruction. The advantage of the use of flushing controlled by real-time imaging is the avoidance of additional lesion caused by forceful blind irrigation. The site of obstruction is described according to anatomical landmarks.

Normally, CM flows freely down the lacrimal system into the nose (Fig. 13.1). In patients with stenosis, early reflux through the punctum with a residual flow of CM to the nasal cavity is seen (Fig. 13.2), in contrast with complete obstruction, when no CM reaches the nasal cavity (Figs. 13.3, 13.4). Furthermore three-dimensional (3D) rotational angiography (3D RA) techniques provide valuable additional information regarding the site and degree of stenotic lesions and the adjacent anatomical structures (Lüchtenberg et al. 2005).

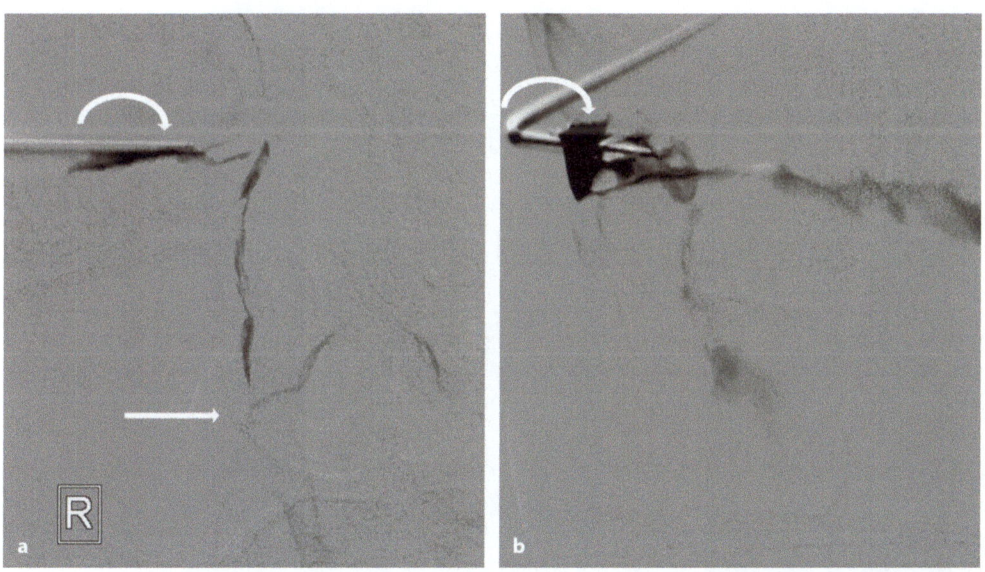

Fig. 13.2. Dacryocystography. Digital subtracted image demonstrates obstruction of the NLDS with reduced contrast medium passage to the nasal cavity (*straight arrow* in **a**) and contrast medium reflux to the eyelid (*curved arrow* in **a, b**). Stenosis of the inferior cannaliculus (frontal view). Additionally (lateral view), the nasolacrimal duct is scarred down with irregularity and focal stenosis at the junction between the nasolacrimal sac and nasolacrimal duct, and at the valve of Hasner. **a** DCG, right-eye frontal view. **b** DCG, right-eye lateral view

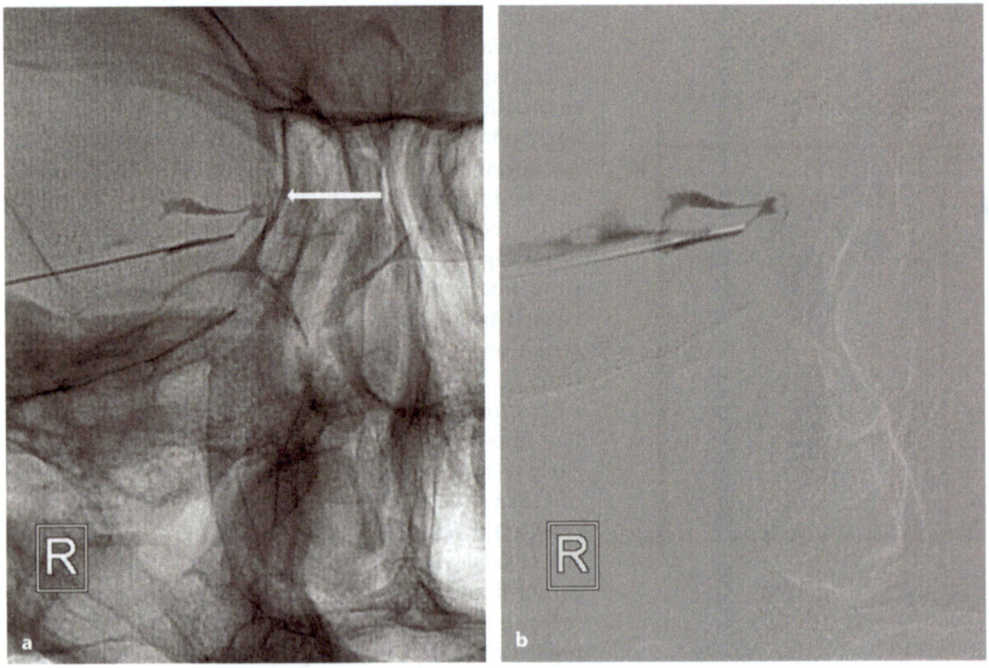

Fig. 13.3. a Dacryocystography, right eye, frontal view. b Digital subtracted image demonstrates complete obstruction of the NLDS at the level of the common cannaliculus (*arrow*)

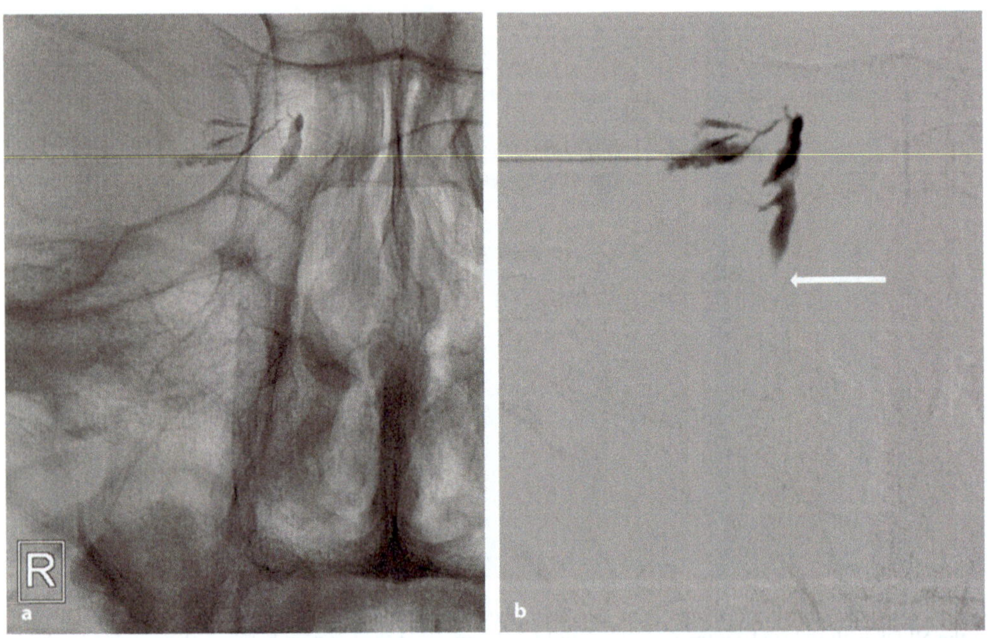

Fig. 13.4. a Dacryocystography, right eye, frontal view. b Digital subtracted image demonstrates complete obstruction of the nasolacrimal duct (*arrow*)

13.2.4 Postoperative Care and Complications: Results

Special postoperative care is not necessary. Besides an allergy against the CM, there are no complications.

In a retrospective analysis of 355 diagnostic dacryocystographies in 281 patients suffering from epiphora, 71% had a tear duct obstruction; in about one-third a stenosis, and in about two-thirds complete obstruction was responsible (Hofer et al. 2000). The stenoses were localized at the junction of saccus and nasolacrimal duct in 31 (38%) cases, postsaccal in 26 (32%) cases, in the common canaliculus in 24 (29%) cases, and rarely (i.e., in 1 case), at the lower canaliculus 1 (1%). The site of complete obstruction was the junction of saccus and nasolacrimal duct in 99 (59%), and the common canaliculus in 29 (17%) cases; it was postsaccal in 27 (16%), and lower canaliculus in 14 (8%) cases; thus, epiphora is mostly caused by stenosis or complete obstruction of the nasolacrimal duct system, with complete obstructions being more frequent than stenoses. The most common site of obstruction is the junction of the saccus and nasolacrimal duct.

13.3 Balloon Dilation

13.3.1 Indications

Especially in cases of incomplete obstruction of the lacrimal system, balloon dilation has become an alternative to surgical procedures in many cases (Janssen et al. 1994; Lee et al. 1994; Song et al. 1996; Wilhelm et al. 1997; Song et al. 2002). In addition, concrements, i.e., dacryoliths of the lacrimal system, which may result from to lacrimal flow obstruction, may be removed or flushed out during the intervention (Wilhelm et al. 1999).

13.3.2 Instrumentation

Lacrimal balloon dilation was first described by Becker and Berry in 1989, followed by Munk et al. in 1990. Becker and Berry introduced a 3- to 4-mm coronary angioplasty catheter through the cannaliculus in an antegrade approach, whereas Munk et al. introduced a 3- to 4-mm tibial angioplasty catheter through the inferior opening of the nasolacrimal duct in a retrograde approach. Meanwhile special low-profile dacryocystoplasty catheters have been designed allowing safe balloon dilation performed antegradely using the transcanalicular access (Wilhelm et al. 2000); therefore, no further nasal manipulation is necessary resulting in greater patient comfort and acceptance of the procedure. We prefer to use 2-mm balloon diameter for obstructions of the canaliculi and 3 mm for obstructions of the nasolacrimal duct and sac. The inflation pressure routinely applied to reach complete balloon inflation is about 10 bar. The duration of inflation of the balloon catheter ranges from 20 min to 15 s (Song 2002). We emphasize that the balloon catheter should be inflated for a short time, to prevent severe damage to the lacrimal drainage system and the surrounding structures, especially the venous plexus (Wilhelm et al. 1999).

13.3.3 Anesthesia

In contrast to most surgical procedures, balloon dilation can be performed as an outpatient procedure under local anesthesia, except in children who do not cooperate with the procedure. The basic interventional procedure consists of the following steps: After local anesthesia of the conjunctival sac by repeated application of two to four drops of oxybuprocainhydrochlorid 0.4% (Novesine 0.4, CIBA Vision Ophthalmics, Germering, Germany), the canaliculi are irrigated with 1–2 ml of the local anesthetic. In addition, anesthesia of the nasal mucosa with oxybuprocainhydrochlorid 1% (Novesine Wander 1%, Wander Pharma, Nürnberg, Germany) may be necessary.

13.3.4 Operative Technique

Under fluoroscopic guidance, a flexible 0.014-in. guidewire (e.g., Skipper, Steerable Guidewire, Invatec, Concesio, Italy) is introduced through the punctum across the obstruction into the inferior meatus of the nasal cavity (Fig. 13.5). The deflated balloon dacryocystoplastycatheter (WAVE, Dacryocystoplasty Balloon Catheter, Invatec, Concesio, Italy) is then advanced antegradely over the wire and positioned across the obstruction. Dilation is performed by inflating the balloon with water-soluble CM. The technical result of dilation is visible under fluoroscopic control immediately. Sufficient widening of

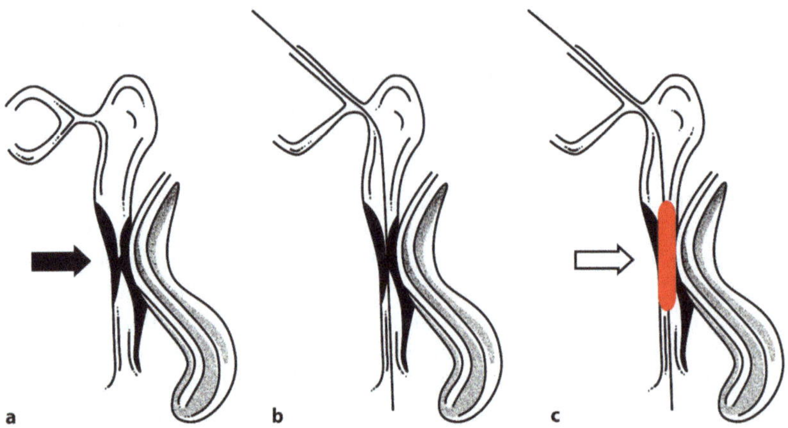

Fig. 13.5. The nasolacrimal duct system (right eye, frontal view) shows incomplete obstruction of the NLDS (*arrow* in a). After recanalization of the stenosis (b), balloon dilation is performed (3-mm balloon diameter; *arrow* in c)

the obstruction is achieved only if the balloon fully opens during inflation. In case of residual obstruction, the balloon will not completely enfold and fluoroscopy shows a residual hourglass deformity (Fig. 13.6). To avoid damage to the lacrimal drainage system after the dilation first the guide wire is removed superiorly, followed by removal of the deflated balloon catheter.

Mild pain during balloon inflation might occur, as might blood-tinged nasal discharge after the procedure. Dacryocystography followed by forced irrigation is performed immediately after the procedure to access the patency of the nasolacrimal duct system.

13.3.5 Postoperative Care and Complications: Results

Postinterventionally the patients are treated with decongestant eyedrops (e.g., Xylometazolinhydrochloride; Otriven, Zyma, Munich, Germany) for at least 1 week (two drops, four to five times a day). Additionally, Refobacin eyedrops (1 ml = 3 mg Gentamicin, Refobacin, Merck, Darmstadt, Germany) are used routinely as topical prophylactic antibiotic therapy. We do not recommend routinely prophylactic oral antibiotics prior to dacryocystoplasty.

Since initial reports by Becker and Berry (1990), several large series have attested to the efficacy of lacrimal balloon dilation. Technical success rates of 89–95% have been reported. According to the experiences of Lee et al. (1994) with 430 eyes of 350 patients, the technical success rate and the overall initial improvement rate were 95 and 57%, respectively. The 2-month, 1-year, and 5-year improvement rates were 48, 39, and 37%, respectively.

This technique can be successfully used in congenital dacryostenosis also (Huenerbein et al 2005). We found a cumulative clinical success rate in 98% after a mean follow-up of 18.4 months in 46 children (mean age 23.5 months).

The technical failure rate and re-obstruction rate is higher in patients with posttraumatic or postsurgical obstructions than in those with idiopathic obstructions. Nevertheless, no major complications have been reported and patient compliance and contentment are very high.

13.4 Stent Placement

13.4.1 Indications

Stent placement is indicated in patients who suffer from epiphora caused by a complete obstruction of the nasolacrimal drainage system and who refuse surgical procedures or are not suitable candidates for general anesthesia. Stent implantation is done in a retrograde fashion using special nasolacrimal duct polyurethane stents.

13.4.2 Instrumentation

In 1994 Song et al. first described fluoroscopic-guided insertion of plastic stents into the nasolacrimal duct as an alternative to surgical procedures. Initially so-called mushroom stents have been used in the treat-

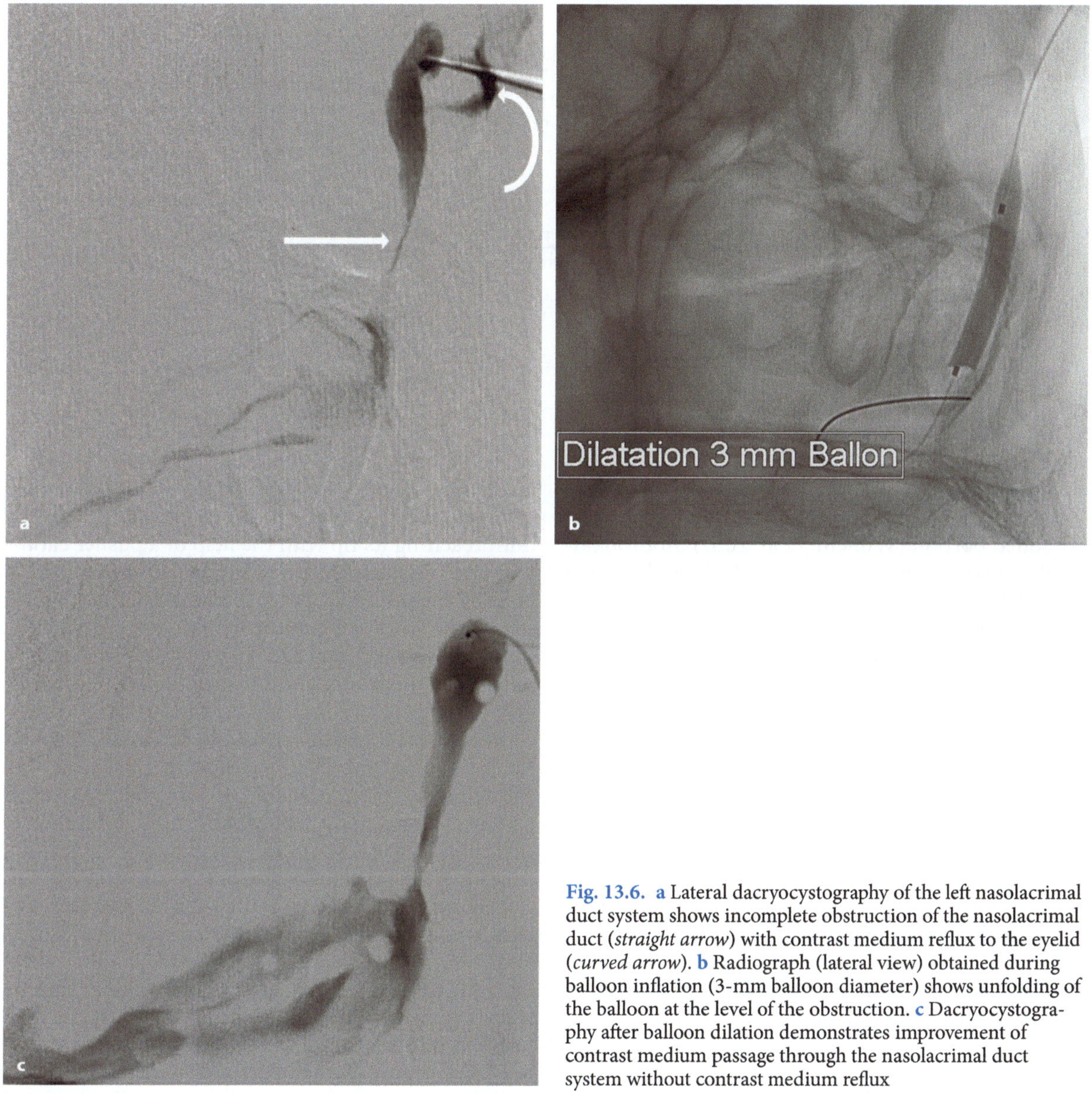

Fig. 13.6. **a** Lateral dacryocystography of the left nasolacrimal duct system shows incomplete obstruction of the nasolacrimal duct (*straight arrow*) with contrast medium reflux to the eyelid (*curved arrow*). **b** Radiograph (lateral view) obtained during balloon inflation (3-mm balloon diameter) shows unfolding of the balloon at the level of the obstruction. **c** Dacryocystography after balloon dilation demonstrates improvement of contrast medium passage through the nasolacrimal duct system without contrast medium reflux

ment of complete obstruction of the lacrimal drainage system. The primary result with these techniques seemed promising (Perena et al. 2001; Song et al. 1996; Wilhelm et al. 1997). Nevertheless, lacrimal stents can be occluded and, in contrast to the excellent technical success rates, the long-time patency rate decreases to 19.2% after follow-up of 5 years (Song et al. 2002). The main problem of the procedure is the tendency towards obstruction of the stent by granulation tissue or mucoid material in the proximal portion of the mushroom stent (Schaudig et al. 2000). To overcome the limitations of the conventional polyurethane stent designed by Song (1994), we designed a new stent type with alterations made in material and stent design (TearLeader Stent with hydrofeel coating, InterV/PBN Medicals, Denmark). This stent is 6 F in

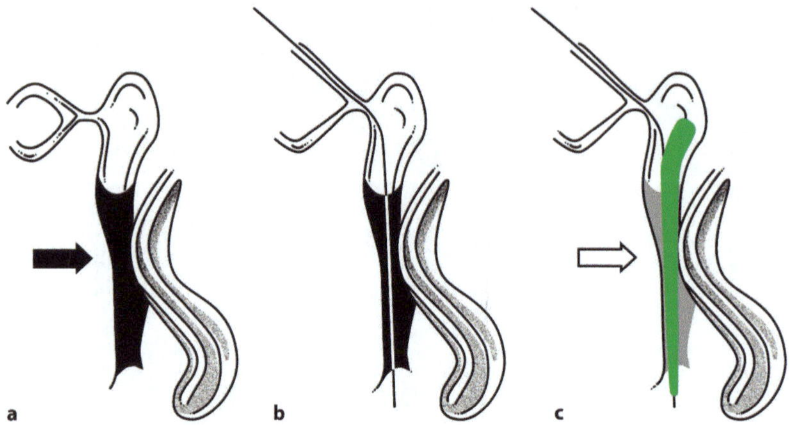

Fig. 13.7. a Drawing of the nasolacrimal duct system (right eye, frontal view) shows complete obstruction of the NLDS (*arrow*). b After recanalization of the stenosis with a guide wire, a polyurethane stent is introduced. c The 6.0 F stent is advanced over the wire until its proximal tapered S-shaped tip is located in the lacrimal sac (*arrow*)

diameter and 35 mm in length. It has a slightly S-shaped configuration and a tapered ending without ballooned portion (Wilhelm et al. 2002). Additionally, the surface of the stent is hydrofeel coated (Fig. 13.7).

The TearLeader stent set consists of a dilator, a stent pusher, a 0.47-mm angled atraumatic nitinol guide wire with a 7-cm hydrophilic radiopaque flexible tip, and a DCG catheter. For diagnostic purposes and to plan the intervention, DCG is performed in posteroanterior and lateral views. Digital subtraction DCG is performed before stent implantation to demonstrate the side of obstruction and to exclude anatomical irregularities and variants.

13.4.3 Anesthesia

Stent placement can be performed on an outpatient basis under local anesthesia.

13.4.4 Operative Technique

The technique for implanting the conventional mushroom stent has been described in detail by Song et al. (1995) several times before: a 0.018-in. ball-tipped guide wire is introduced into the nasolacrimal duct system and gently advanced until reaching the inferior meatus of the nasal cavity. It is pulled out of the external naris with a hook. Then a 6.3-F nasolacrimal sheath with a tapered dilator is passed retrogradely over the guide wire subsequently into the upper part of the nasolacrimal system (Fig. 13.8). The dilator is removed and the stent is introduced into the sheath until reaching its tip with the help of a pusher catheter. After this, the sheath has to be withdrawn while holding the pusher catheter in place, thus freeing the stent and allowing the mushroom tip to expand within the dilated lacrimal sac. Finally, the guide wire is pulled out superiorly and the pusher catheter inferiorly.

In contrast to these mushroom stents, the method for implanting the TearLeader stent (Fig. 13.9) was simplified to improve the procedure and to advance patients comfort: the most important difference is that no additional sheath for introducing the stent is necessary thanks to its well-tapered stent ending. The first step of the procedure is to probe the nasolacrimal duct system with a DCG catheter. Then a flexible-angled nitinol guide wire is introduced via the catheter into the nasolacrimal duct system. Under fluoroscopic guidance the guide wire is gently pushed forward into the inferior meatus of the nasal cavity until protruding from the external naris.

Before stent implantation, the specially designed tapered DCG catheter from the stent set has to be advanced anterogradely over the guide wire until leaving the nostril as well. From distal position the stent is threaded on the guide wire directly followed by a stent pusher. Next step the stent and the stent pusher have to be retrogradely advanced over the guide wire until making contact with the DCG catheter. Carefully fixing the anastomosis of DCG catheter (proximal), stent, and stent pusher (distal) to the guide wire, the stent is now brought into position under fluoroscopic

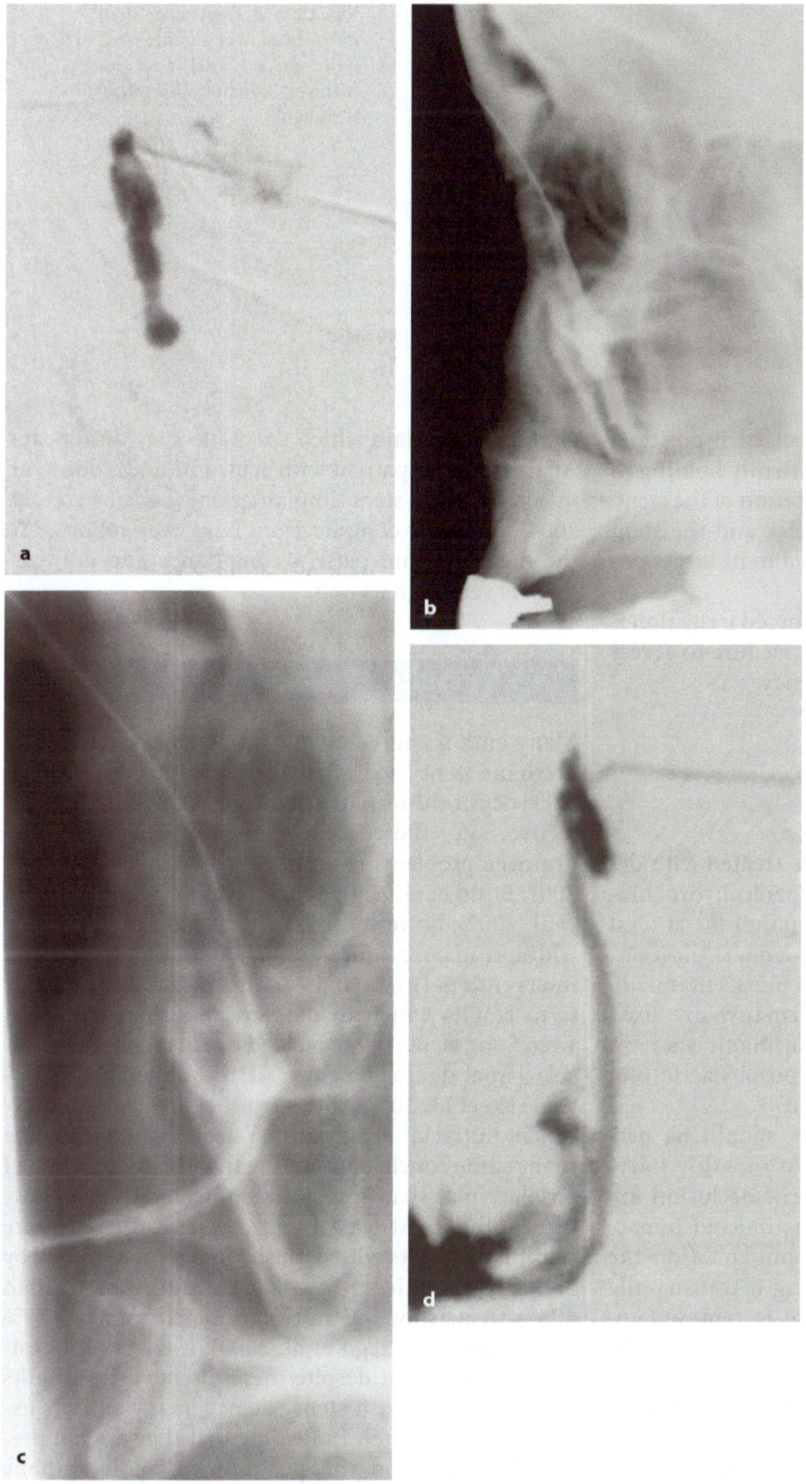

Fig. 13.8. a Dacryocystography (frontal view) shows complete obstruction of the left nasolacrimal duct system (a). b Radiograph (lateral view) obtained after recanalization of the obstruction demonstrates a 0.018 in. ball-tipped guide wire which is introduced into the nasolacrimal duct system and gently advanced until reaching the inferior meatus of the nasal cavity (b). c Stent implantation (lateral view): From distal the stent retrogradely advanced over the guide wire until correct position of the stent is achieved. d Dacryocystography after stent implantation shows a patent stent with contrast medium passage through the stent into the inferior meatus of the nasal cavity

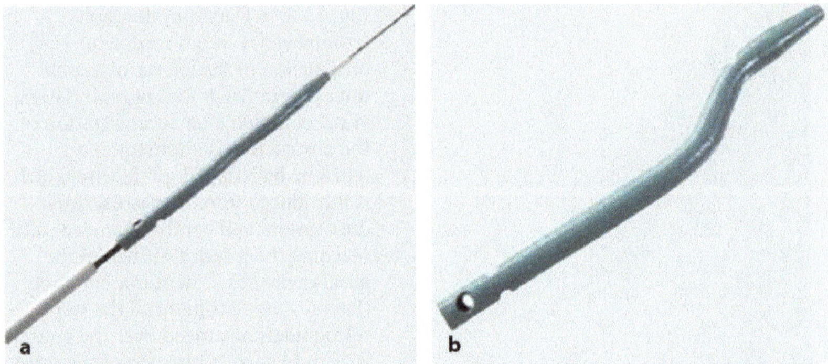

Fig. 13.9. a TearLeader stent introduced over a guide wire. **b** Pre-shaped TearLeader stent with two side holes for retrieval is shown

control. After having reached correct stent position, the guide wire is pulled back while firmly holding in place the stent pusher to avoid dislocation of the stent. Then, the dacryocystography catheter and the stent pusher are retracted, leaving the stent in its target position.

Dacryocystography followed by forced irrigation is performed immediately after the procedure to access correct stent position and stent patency.

13.4.5 Postoperative Care and Complications

Postinterventionally the patients are treated with decongestant eyedrops (e.g., Xylometazolinhydrochloride; Otriven, Zyma, Munich, Germany) for at least 1 week (two drops, four to five times a day). Additionally, Refobacin eyedrops (1 ml = 3 mg Gentamicin, Refobacin, Merck, Darmstadt, Germany) are used routinely as topical prophylactic antibiotic therapy. We do not recommend routinely prophylactic oral antibiotics prior to stent implanation.

Clinical follow-up examinations should be performed at intervals of 1 week, and at monthly intervals thereafter. The reasons for stent occlusion are usually granulation tissue as well as mucoid impactions in the stent. Two months after implantation, the stent should be removed by grasping it transnasally with a hook or forceps. Rarely, it has to removed endoscopically when it cannot be grasped, or when tight granulation tissue holds it in place.

During stent implantation mild pain sensation might occur, as might blood-tinged nasal discharge after the procedure. Commonly the patients report from a foreign-body sensation at the medial cantal region for a few days which spontaneously disappears. Apart from one patient with acute blindness due to an infection after stent implantation (Lanciego et al. 2004), no major complications have been reported in the literature and patient compliance and contentment is very high as well.

13.5 Results

Many authors agree on the attractiveness of a polyurethane stent used as an alternative to conventional dacryocystorhinostomy because it offers an easy, effective, safe, and reversible way to manage lacrimal drainage problems (Kang et al. 2002; Lanciego et al. 2001; Pinto et al. 2001; Schaudig et al. 2000; Wilhelm et al. 2002); however, this method has not yet gained widespread acceptance among ophthalmologists and interventional radiologists. This is due to the long-term results which to date are less than favorable. Even Song et al. (1995) decided not to recommend nasolacrimal duct stents as a first-line therapeutic option (Ko et al. 2003), although they had achieved excellent initial clinical results. Yazici et al. (2002) came to the same conclusion, stating that the success rate of nasolacrimal stent implantation decreases as follow-up lengthens. At least Laciego et al. gathered more optimistic results with a mushroom stent designed by Song in a multicentric study recruiting more than 400 patients showing a primary patency rate of 59% after 5 years (Laciego et al. 2003). It is very interesting, however, that despite these discouraging results regarding long-term stent patency, many authors express a point of view indicating that they are not prepared to abandon the possibility of polyurethane stenting in tear-duct obstructions straight away.

Schaudig and Maas (2005), for example, admit that the overall success rate is lower than that reported after conventional dacryocystorhinostomy, yet they draw the conclusion that refinement of the surface and stent design may improve results in the future.

The short-term observation after implantation of the newly designed hydrophilicly coated TearLeader stent has already shown a clear tendency towards more favorable results. This also includes the good feasibility and greater patient comfort during the implantation procedure, as has been shown in our studies (Wilhelm et al. 2003) and in the first long-term clinical results reported by Ferrer-Puchol et al. (Ferrer-Puchol et al. 2000); however, longer follow-up periods will be required to define the role of stent implantation finally.

13.6 Highlights

Advances in interventional techniques in the lacrimal drainage system have expanded novel procedures for the easy and safe treatment of epiphora. These methods are simple, safe, and cost-effective, and can be performed under local anesthesia on an outpatient basis. They cause no facial scars and fewer problems with bleeding, resulting in less postoperative complications with high patient compliance and contentment.

Fluoroscopically guided balloon dacryocystoplasty is a feasible nonsurgical therapy in nasolacrimal duct stenosis that may be used as first-line therapy. In cases that have initial success, however, a relatively high long-term success rate can be expected.

Stent placement should be selected with caution as a first-line therapeutic option in patients who refuse surgical procedures or are not suitable to general anesthesia. Although the initial results of stent placement in patients with complete obstructions of the lacrimal drainage system are excellent, long-term results have to be improved.

Reference

Becker BB, Berry FD. Balloon catheter dilation in lacrimal surgery. Ophthalmic Surg 1989;20:193–198

Ewing AE. Roentgen ray demonstration of the lacrimal abscess cavity. Am J Ophthalmol 1989;26:1–4

Ferrer-Puchol M, Esteban-Hernández E, Jornet-Frayos J, Ferragus-Gibes S, Sanifélix-Micó P, Terol-Penalva D (2005) Obstruction of the lacrimal system. Treatment and long term results with polyurethane Song stent versus Tear Leader-Stent. Annual Meeting and Postgraduate Course of the Cardiovascular and Interventional Radiological Society of Europe, Abstract Book Poster 30, 164

Hofer U, Wilhelm KE, Loeffler K, Schild H. Diagnostic Digital-Subtraction-Dacryozystography: Technique, Criteria of Evaluation, Frequency and Localization of Pathological Findings. Radiology 2000;217(P):223

Huenerbein R, Grass F, Leber M, Wilhelm K, Kuhn FP. Balloon dacryocystoplasty: interventional radiological therapy of congenital dacryostenosis. Rofo 2005; 177:1387–1393

Janssen AG, Mansour K, Rabbe GJ. Dacryocystoplasty: treatment of epiphora by means of ballon dilation of the obstructed nasolacrimal duct system. Radiology 1994;193:453–456

Kang SG, Song HY, Lee DH, Choi JY, Ahn HS. Nonsurgically placed nasolacrimal stents for epiphora: long-term results and factors favoring stent patency. J Vasc Interv Radiol 2002;13:293–300

Kassel EE, Schatz CJ. Lacrimal Apparatus. In: Som PM, Curtin HD (eds) Head and neck imaging, 3rd edn. Mosby, St. Louis, 1995;1129–1183

Ko GY, Song HY et al. Obstruction of the lacrimal system: treatment with a covered, retrievable, expandable nitinol stent versus a lacrimal polyurethane stent. Radiology 2003;227:270–276

Lanciego C, Miguel S de, Perea M et al. Nasolacrimal stents in the management of epiphora: medium-term results of a multicenter prospective study. J Vasc Interv Radiol 2001;12:701–710

Lanciego C, Toledano N et al. Resolution of epiphora with nasolacrimal stents: results of long-term follow-up in a multicenter prospective study. J Vasc Interv Radiol 2003;14:1417–1425

Lanciego C, Bracamonte A, Mendez-Cendon JC, Gomez C, Padilla M, Garcia-Garcia L. Loss of vision as a complication of nasolacrimal stent placement. J Vasc Interv Radiol 2004;15:1027–1028

Lee JM, Song HY, Han YM, Chung GH, Sohn MH, Kim KS, Choi KC. Balloon dacryocystoplasty. Results in the treatment of complete and partial obstructions of the nasolacrimal system. Radiology 1994;192:503–508

Lüchtenberg M, Kuhli C et al. Three-dimensional rotational dacryocystography for imaging of the lacrimal drainage system and adjacent anatomical structures. Ophthalmologia 2005; 219:136–141

Munk PL, Lin DTC, Morris DC. Epiphora: treatment by means of dacryocystoplasty with balloon dilation of the nasolacrimal drainage apparatus. Radiology 1990;177:687–690

Perena MF, Castillo J, Medrano J, Gregorio MA de, Loras E, Cristobal JA. Nasolacrimal polyurethane stent placement: preliminary results. Eur J Ophthalmol 2001;11:25–30

Pinto I, Paul L, Grande C, Cal MA de la. Nasolacrimal polyurethane stent placement for epiphora: technical long-term results. J Vasc Interv Radiol 2001;12:67–71

Schaudig U, Maas R. The polyurethane nasolacrimal duct stent for lower tear duct obstruction: long-term success rate and complications. Graefes Arch Clin Exp Ophthalmol 2000;238:733–737

Song HY, Jin HY, Kim JH, Sung KB, Han YM, Cho NC. Nasolacrimal duct obstruction treated nonsurgically with use of plastic stents. Radiology 1994;190:535–539

Song HY, Jin Y-H, Kim J-H, Huh S-J, Kim Y-H, Kom T-H, Sung K-B. Nonsurgical placement of a nasolacrimal polyurethane stent. Radiology 1995;194:233–237

Song HY et al. Non-surgical placement of a nasolacrimal polyurethane stent: long-term effectiveness. Radiology 1996;200:759–763

Song, H-Y, Lee DH, Ahn H, Seo T-S, Ko G-Y. Intervention in the lacrimal drainage system. Cardiovasc Intervent Radiol 2002;25:165–170

Wilhelm K, Textor J, Hofer U, Böker T, Strunk H, Schild H. Nasolacrimal duct obstructions: treatment with balloon dilation and stent implantation. Fortschr Röntgenstr 1997;167:486–490

Wilhelm K, Hofer U, Textor J, Böker T, Strunk H, Schild H. Nonsurgical fluoroscopically guided treatment of dacryoliths during dacrycystoplasty. Radiology 1999:212:365–370

Wilhelm K, Hofer U, Textor HJ, Böker T, Strunk H, Schild HH. Nonsurgical fluoroscopically guided dacryocystoplasty of common canalicular obstructions. Cardiovasc Intervent Radiol 2000;23:1–8

Wilhelm KE, Hofer U, Textor J, Loeffler K, Urbach H, Schild HH. Antegrade transcanalicular dacryocystoplasty of nasolacrimal duct obstructions. Radiology 2000;217(P):324

Wilhelm K, Loeffler K, Urbach H, Schild H. Complete tear duct obstruction: treatment with lacrimal polyurethane stent implantation. Cardiovasc Intervent Radiol 2002;25: S149

Wilhelm K, Loeffler K, Urbach H, Schild H. Behandlung von Tränenwegsverschlüssen mit dem PBN Wilhelm TearLeader Stent: Erste Ergebnisse. Fortschr Röntgenstr 2003;175 S1:152–153

Yazici Z, Yazici B, Parlak M, Tuncel E, Ertürk H. Treatment of nasolacrimal duct obstruction with polyurethane stent placement: long-term results. AJR 2002;179:491–494

Subject Index

MIX
Papier aus verantwortungsvollen Quellen
Paper from responsible sources
FSC® C105338

If you have any concerns about our products,
you can contact us on
ProductSafety@springernature.com

In case Publisher is established outside the EU,
the EU authorized representative is:
Springer Nature Customer Service Center GmbH
Europaplatz 3, 69115 Heidelberg, Germany

Printed by Libri Plureos GmbH
in Hamburg, Germany